First published in Great Britain in 2002 by
Arnold, a member of the Hodder Headline Group
338 Euston Road, London NW1 3BH

http://www.arnoldpublishers.com

Distributed in the United States of America by
Oxford University Press Inc.,
198 Madison Avenue, New York, NY 10016

British Library Cataloguing in Publication Data
A catalogue record for this book is available from the British Library

Library of Congress Cataloging-in-Publication Data
A catalog record for this book is available from the Library of Congress

ISBN 0 340 75971 2

2 3 4 5 6 7 8 9 10

Typeset in 10 on 12 Sabon by Phoenix Photosetting, Chatham, Kent
Printed and bound in Malta by Gutenberg Press Ltd

What do you think about this book? Or any other Arnold title?
Please send your comments to feedback.arnold@hodder.co.uk

Essential Health Psychology

Mark Forshaw

Senior Lecturer in Psychology, Coventry University, UK
Chartered Health Psychologist

A
ARNOLD

A member of the Hodder Headline Group
LONDON

Distributed in the United States of America by
Oxford University Press Inc., New York

Contents

Preface

This book will not tell you everything you want to know about health psychology. I know of no book, in my opinion, which can. (If it were the case, you would only need the one book, and all others would be worthless.) You will not find a discussion of every topic that health psychology involves. It is a short book, an introduction. I have not packed the book with reference after reference to studies. I have opted, instead, for a much lighter touch. I have chosen to explain, in beginners' terms, some basic concepts which form the essence of health psychology today. The often discursive style is part of a deliberate approach aimed at opening up an area of considerable academic merit and sophistication to people who are encountering it for the first time. They might be psychologists in the making, or nurses or doctors, physio-therapists, occupational therapists, training or practising. They might have no knowledge of health issues, or they might have considerable expertise but are interested in what psychology has to offer them.

I have succeeded in my aim if you read this book and want to read more about health psychology. Computers are tremendously complicated machines that can do impressive things. But, at first you have to press a button to start them up. It is only one little button, and it only requires one little push, but it is the first step in something much bigger and better and quite fascinating. This book, I hope, is like that button.

(I cannot operate in isolation. A number of people have assisted me, in a variety of ways, in producing this book. I have thanked them personally for it, and simply reiterate it here. Thank you, everyone.)

Dr Mark Forshaw
January 2002

1 Introduction

Health psychology is a term made up of two words which are both almost impossible to define. Look in ten books on health and each will define it differently. Look in ten books on psychology and the same problem will occur. This will be more noticeable if the books come from different decades, since the meanings of these words keep on changing over time. It is probably safest if we plump for the widest possible definitions of each. For the purposes of this book, health is the state where a person functions, physically and mentally, efficiently and effectively with relative comfort and a sense of well-being. Psychology is the study of the psyche. That is, psychology is the study of human thought, feeling and behaviour. Health psychology, therefore, is loosely definable as the study of how thoughts, feelings and behaviours stem from, interact with, or cause, physical or mental efficiency, efficacy, comfort and well-being.

Health psychology is a relatively new branch of psychology, which is, in itself, a relatively new sphere of study, little older than a century. Health psychology was unheard of until the 1970s. When it first appeared it was often called medical psychology, or, when it was taught in undergraduate medical programmes, it sometimes fell under the heading of 'behavioural medicine'. Today, health psychology is not just an area of academic study, but, depending upon the country you are in, it is a profession.

Health psychology is not just of interest to psychologists, but also to anyone interested in human health and illness. Health psychologists endeavour to discover why people behave in the ways that they do which endanger their health. They work on achieving ways in which information can be provided to promote health so that people understand it, remember it, and act on it. Health psychologists do not, generally, deal with mental illness, and certainly never seek to 'cure' it directly. That is the purpose of clinical psychology and psychiatry. However, as Bennett (2000) admits, at times the demarcations between health psychology and clinical psychology are far from clear, and debate continues. Psychologists' professional bodies continue in their endeavours to promote health psychology and to establish it as an unequivocally recognised complement to hospital services, in addition to being a clearly defined academic discipline. Some people argue that health psychology should be only the academic study of health, others that health psychologists have practical skills to offer. This debate continues.

Largely, health psychologists study groups of people to generalise their findings to other groups. They look for personality types which underpin behaviours, and they seek to explain things by producing models of what happens when and why and to whom. They experiment, they observe, they interview, they survey, they test. Reading this book should give you a strong sense of what psychologists have to offer to the study of health and illness.

Of course, not all health psychology need be, or indeed is, focused on groups and the behaviour of types or classes of people. Equally it can be about individuals, and their very idiosyncratic health problems. Psychologists, on the whole, have an equal interest in the nomothetic and idiographic approaches to the study of human behaviour. The nomothetic approach concerns groups, and the idiographic stance looks at behaviour at the level of the individual. Particular psychologists have preferences for one over the other, just as they may have preferences for quantitative research over qualitative, but in the discipline itself both approaches are very well represented. You will find, in your reading, that health psychologists often have to be quite eclectic, turning to other disciplines like sociology at times. Health psychologists cannot ignore inequalities in health, for instance. If someone lives in a culture where sugary foodstuffs are valued, a financially poor culture which means that they also cannot afford to pay for their teeth to be regularly examined and repaired by a dentist, it might explain why they have poor dental health. It also might explain why they do not seem to place a great deal of value on having clean, strong teeth. There is no point in developing long-winded psychological models when the sociological model explains most of the behaviour. Health psychologists must be open to studying the range of things that affect a person's health status, without losing sense of the specific contribution that a psychologist can make to discourses on health. Do not be surprised, therefore, if sometimes you read in health psychology literature (including this book) about things said by sociologists, health scientists, medical anthropologists, health lawyers, and the like. A good health psychologist does not ignore information from any source provided that it may be useful to them in working out what is going on in a person's mind which can determine how they think about their body and how they treat it.

The work of health psychologists is not easy. The world is a complicated place, and people are the most unfathomable things in it. Scientists are just beginning to discover the unpredictability that there is in the universe. Chaos theory is in its infancy. We are told of the butterfly flapping its wings which, through a sequence of events, causes an earthquake thousands of miles away. Individual people can be affected in significant ways by seemingly trivial events in their lives, or the lives of others which then impinge on theirs. People are influenced by their upbringing, by their peers, by their financial status, by whims, by ambition, by culture, by society, by law, by random events which occur, by plans they have which may or may not be foiled, and sometimes, seemingly, by nothing at all. When a psychologist undertakes to discover why someone does something, they take on the world in all its complexity.

In a sense, this is not unlike a view that both top-down and bottom-up processes can affect an outcome. Health psychology, like all psychology, should, ideally, concern itself with both top-down and bottom-up explanations of phenomena. For an example outside of health, there are generally two ways in which a person can have strong religious faith. They might have been raised in a strongly religious family and community. Their sense of spirituality may have developed vicariously, and to some extent have been handed down from people around them. So, they start with a view that there is a divine presence, and so they then view the world in terms of that 'truth' for them. This would be top-down processing. Some people, however, 'discover' their faith. They start off with no strong belief, and develop a sense of spirituality from the things around them. As you will have heard, people see the world, mountains, flowers, and so on, and 'feel' a sense of divine purpose 'speaking' to them this way. This creation of a sense of a god or gods from little things added together could be said to be a form of bottom-up processing. Each one is important in its own right, and neither is specifically the right way to view things. If we take an example from health now, if we were trying to predict a person's chances of having a heart attack then a top-down health psychology approach might look for evidence of a prone personality (see Types A and B personality via the Index for details). The bottom-up approach would look for behavioural concomitants of heart disease such as exercise patterns, stress, diet, smoking behaviour and so on. Of course, the good health psychologist looks both ways at once. A combination of what might be called endogenous and exogenous factors (or intrinsic/extrinsic, internal/external) will, in reality, determine if a person develops heart disease and is subject to an infarction. Looking one way only, if you are crossing the road, can be very dangerous. Researchers need to be just as vigilant.

In a sense, health psychology is about understanding needs, and how people seek to satisfy their needs. Early work by Maslow (1962) identified a 'hierarchy of needs' that the human organism has. Some are more basic than others, and therefore are prioritised when the person tries to reduce their environmental stresses by satisfying their needs. Food and drink are the first rung on this ladder of requirements. Then comes the requirement for the organism to feel safe. Further up this hierarchy are more subtle human requirements such as the need to be liked by peers and to be loved. Then, above this is the more subtle need for esteem. Satisfying all needs is necessary for the highest level of well-being possible for the individual. Unmet needs cause strain upon the individual. You can probably see how closely health-related behaviours can be mapped onto this framework. Many health-supporting and health-injurious behaviours are underpinned by needs from this hierarchy. As you will learn from this book, health psychology is partly concerned with

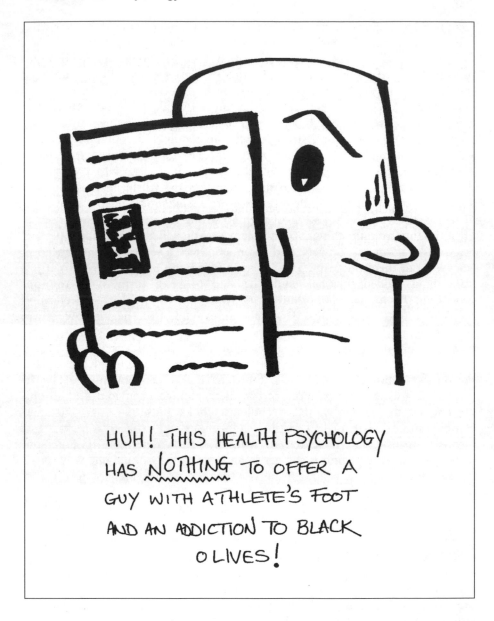

appetitive behaviour: people eating too little or too much, smoking, engaging in harmful sexual practices, and so on. In doing these things, they are working to satisfy needs in Maslow's hierarchy. That is probably why health psychologists might always be required; there will always be human beings spurred on by fundamental drives to perform acts which, ultimately, are damaging to them.

MODELS

Health psychology is driven largely by the **biopsychosocial model** of health and illness. It arose partly as a reaction to the older, prevailing **medical model**. The medical model is based upon a centuries-old conception of science and the view that there is a truth to be assessed and recorded. This is known as positivism. It still drives most science today, and indeed a great deal of modern psychology is positivistic in nature. There is reductionism, or the view that eventually all phenomena can be explained by recourse to describing chemicals, cells and processes. There is also an inherent mind–body dualism, that is the mind and the body are seen as separate things to be studied and assessed as such. The concept of mind–body dualism is such a distinct characteristic of the medical model, but is conspicuously lacking in Eastern medical systems such as Chinese medicine. Traditional Chinese doctors are interested in the whole person, and would never make a diagnosis without learning something about the person, their likes and dislikes, habits, behaviours, and personality. They believe, probably quite rightly as evidence from health psychology shows, that all of these things create the health status of a person, not just what is happening to their body on a fundamental level. Interestingly enough, this holistic view is what is fundamental to the biopsychosocial model of health and illness. Most health psychologists accept that people are biological organisms, and that their biology can determine a lot of their behaviours, but also realise that thoughts and feelings can have a significant influence upon what a person does and does not do. The medical model became increasingly outmoded as we began to generate more and more questions which it could not provide answers for. A model which ignores the individual, which ignores culture, society, religion, individual differences in personality and cognition and emotion is never going to be able to answer questions like 'Why do teenagers take up smoking?' and 'How stressful is divorce?' The biopsychosocial model is a framework for answering such questions, with its emphasis on understanding the person in the context of their life, whilst not losing sight of the biological underpinnings of our existence.

METHODS

Finally, a word about research methods. Since its beginnings, psychology has been haunted by debates over the most appropriate ways to find things out. In a way, the argument, at times heated, over quantitative versus qualitative methods, reflects individual differences in style and temperament. Some people prefer numbers, some people prefer words. Some people think that interviews tell us most about people, some people think that numerical data (reaction times, test scores and so on) are supremely informative and reliable. There was a time when it was not difficult to find a psychologist who would say that anything other than a controlled experiment was not 'proper' psychology. Interviews and surveys and the like were seen as subjective exercises which had no place in the discipline, especially when the analysis performed was done at the level of the discourse, rather than by counting up or calculating. Equally, there were those people who took a strong stance against all of this, claiming equally vehemently that all quantitative methods were too much driven by the unattainable ideal of objectivity and, ultimately, were the very worst way to explore human behaviour.

There has been a preponderance of quantitative methods over qualitative in psychology since psychology developed from philosophy and needed to make a clear distinction between itself and its forbears. In the last 20 years there has been a marked increase in interest in qualitative methods in psychology, and this is reflected in health psychology too (for example, in the publication of books such as that on qualitative approaches to health psychology edited by Murray and Chamberlain, 1999). Whilst most psychology is still about experimentation and the collection of 'scores', talking to people to find things out is by no means a minority activity any more. Increasingly, psychologists are dedicating themselves to neither camp, but embracing both schools of research. A future where people use a range of means to achieve an end promises to be an exciting one, and perhaps one where more things are found out than ever before.

In this book, you will read about many approaches to solving the puzzles of human health-related behaviour. You will not find any suggestions that one kind of research is better than another, just as you will not find any suggestions that one lifestyle is better than another. The human world is about choice, and psychologists not only study the choices which people make, but make choices of their own, such as how to do research, and whether to find value in the researches of others. Health psychologists today need an open mind if they are to understand the behaviours and motivations of others and if they are to make a difference to the world. To make a journey from A to B, a car needs fuel. The tank cannot be filled unless the fuel cap is taken off.

2 The Biology of Health and Illness

INTRODUCTION

One of the most important lessons that anyone who studies health psychology must learn is that the human body interacts with the mind, and that the two work together to create the overall 'system' which we think of as a person. The physical condition of the body can have a profound impact on the mental state of the person, and the mental state of the person can create new physical states or modify existing ones. People who develop cancer, for example, react to it, and their behaviours, opinions and beliefs, about themselves and the world around them, can all change, to a greater or a lesser extent. If someone is injured in an accident, and their looks change, so might their feelings about themselves. Similarly, a person prone to worrying about things, often when there is no need to worry, can create very real physical problems for themselves, such as headaches, nausea, stomach ulcers, skin conditions, or even heart disease.

A *psychosomatic* illness is one which may be psychological or organic in origin but which usually involves some interaction between the physical and the mental. An illness is said to be *psychogenic* if there is no physical cause, i.e. if it is assumed to be solely psychological in origin. A good example of this is the majority of cases of erectile dysfunction (previously called impotence). If a man is able to have erections first thing in the morning, or in response to friction from clothing, or when masturbating, but not when engaging in sexual activity with another person, the assumption must be that there can be no *physical* impairment. This, therefore, is a psychogenic problem. There is overlap between the two terms although they have subtly different meanings. Different writers and health professionals use the terms with some degree of confusion, and so the above definitions are not hard-and-fast.

It is sometimes theoretically useful to distinguish between three principal categories of psychosomatic disorder. These are: **lifestyle-based** (i.e. where what a person does can affect their health), **personality-based** (where the type of person that someone is seems to engender certain health problems) and **reaction-based** (where a person's reaction to something can create problems). In the case of lifestyle-based disorders, a person may develop a health problem such as heart disease because they have a stressful occupation or choose to eat fatty foods. A high proportion of people would develop the same problem if they lived the same kind of life. However, in the case of personality-based disorders, lifestyle is less important than the characteristics of the individual concerned. Some people are simply more nervous or anxious than others. There is evidence to suggest that this may be because of a mixture of nature and nurture. If nervousness is a property of the nervous system then it could be inherited. Equally, a person raised amongst nervous or anxious people may well learn various behaviours and world-views which make them nervous and anxious too. Anxious people may be more likely to develop heart disease, even when they seem to live relatively stress-free lives, because they might tend to interpret pleasant events as neutral, neutral events as stressful, and stressful events as even more stressful. Reaction-based disorders can often be confused with personality-based ones, and the difference is often negligible or even undetectable. One of the least arguable cases of a reaction-based disorder is something like an allergic reaction which has behavioural consequences, i.e. where a person becomes irritable or violent after consuming certain substances. Of course, these three categories are rarely independent. It is extremely difficult to diagnose based on these divisions, since every person has a personality, a lifestyle, and various reactions to various substances. Without knowing every last detail of a person's life, every aspect of their lifestyle, every facet of their personality, every nuance of their biological makeup, it is virtually impossible to claim that a disorder is entirely personality-based, or entirely reaction-based, or of a mixed aetiology. Like most things in life, health and illness are multivariate: lots of things can create and modify them.

So, a good student of health psychology should be aware of this interplay between mind and body. They are not separate things, and so it does not really make sense to study behaviour unless we study the body too. In this sense, health psychology overlaps with the study of human biology.

'SYSTEMS'

Mainly for the sake of simplicity, the human body is often divided into systems. Some of the main systems of interest to psychologists are mentioned in this chapter. It is important to remember, however, that these systems are at times arbitrary divisions of one bigger system, the body. Exactly where the lines are drawn between systems, and which organs and tissues are in which system, are arguable. Indeed, some structures are in more than one system; the testes and ovaries are both reproductive organs *and* endocrine glands. We divide this way mainly for convenience. Most of the systems feed directly into the others, and a disease or injury in one area can often create problems in others. At times, this categorisation is very useful, but it can also be very artificial. Imagine dividing up a street into the lighting system, the road system and the housing system, for example. Each one can be considered separately. For example, one could study the lighting without thinking too much about the housing, or one could be interested in the way the road was constructed without too much consideration for the lighting. However, anything but the most simplistic focus on these would show that all three work together. Once the sun has gone down, traffic accidents ensue without lighting. The roads have traffic on them partly because of the people coming and going from their houses. The people in the houses like their street to be lit at night, but no-one wants a street light so close to their bedroom window that they cannot sleep (even if it might be beneficial to motorists). The motorists might prefer a straight road, but one might have to be built that bypasses the houses. This book consists of chapters, sections, paragraphs, sentences, words and letters. Studying the letters might mean missing out on some interesting words, and it would be impossible to take in the paragraphs without absorbing the sentences, words and letters. This does not mean that analysis at any given level is not useful or ever appropriate, simply that we must not lose sight of the interrelatedness of things, the blurring of cause and effect within our systems. However one examines each system, the functioning of it depends on the others. The human body is like that. This is partly what makes doctors' jobs so difficult at times (consultants specialise in *one* of the systems, hence we have endocrinology, respiratory medicine, cardiology and so on). It is also why psychologists can be very frustrated when they attempt to pin down a particular behaviour to a particular reason. It is always best to be wary of statements like 'people smoke because they want something to do with their hands' and 'overeating is learned in childhood'. Both statements are probably true to some extent some of the time, but are not accurate to the exclusion of all other variables and hypotheses. Things happen for many reasons, and rarely for one reason alone.

THE ENDOCRINE SYSTEM

Glands which produce hormones are called endocrine glands. Much of our behaviour occurs in some part because of hormones circulating in our bodies which have particular effects, not only on tissues all over the body but specifically in the brain itself. Hormones are chemicals which regulate processes within the body. They are responsible for hunger, thirst, sexual appetites, and so on. If you alter the body's hormonal content, you create, in many respects, a different *person*. To an extent, health psychologists focus on personalities and cognitions and emotions associated with those personalities.

The endocrine system includes the following structures; the hypothalamus, the pineal and pituitary glands, the thyroid, the liver, kidney, pancreas and adrenal gland, the ovaries and the testes. Without hormones, many necessary, normal functions and activities would not occur, such as growth during the lifespan, sexual maturation and so on, but when hormonal levels are changed illness and unusual behaviour can result. Hormonal levels may change because of *endogenous* or *exogenous* factors.

Endogenous factors are things originating *within* the body. For instance, a tumour in the pituitary gland might affect the production of TSH (thyroid-stimulating hormone). This would then affect the amount of thyroxine produced by the thyroid gland in the neck. As a result, a person might suffer from an underactive or overactive thyroid (known as *hypothyroidism* and *hyperthyroidism* respectively). Both of these affect behaviour. In the case of hypothyroidism (also called myxoedema) a lack of thyroxine can lead to sluggishness, weight gain, deepening of the voice and slowness of speech. Hyperthyroidism (thyrotoxicosis) is caused by too much thyroxine circulating in the body. Amongst other things, the person loses weight, their heart beats faster, and they appear agitated and anxious. They can even become noticeably more aggressive. In both cases, the changes in behaviour are enough for people to notice that the person is not 'being themselves'; they are behaving differently.

Exogenous factors originate *outside* of the body. Certain toxins, for example, would be considered exogenous causes. Chronic (long-term) alcohol poisoning can lead to cirrhosis (degeneration) of the liver. This in turn can cause atrophy (shrinkage) of the testes. A consequence of this is infertility. Since the testicles produce the androgen testosterone (a hormone) which is responsible for 'masculine' sexual characteristics, diminishing production of testosterone can create erectile dysfunction and a loss of libido.

THE REPRODUCTIVE SYSTEM

In males, this includes the penis and testicles, and in females the vagina, uterus, Fallopian tubes and ovaries. Health psychologists have made significant inroads into the study of sexual health, and work with health promotors and educators in helping to change attitudes and behaviours which might put individuals at risk from sexually transmitted diseases such as syphilis and AIDS. In addition, attention has been focused onto the ways in which the system can be affected by behaviour and the ways in which the system may malfunction, thus affecting behaviour itself.

Diabetes is a disorder of the endocrine system. However, it can have effects on the reproductive system, such as erectile dysfunction in males. Obviously, erectile dysfunction has the propensity for being a considerable disability for a man. It may have serious consequences for his self-esteem, and his relationships. This may create stress for him. Of course, stress exacts a toll on the cardiovascular system. This, therefore, provides another example of the interrelatedness of the different systems within the body.

THE DIGESTIVE AND EXCRETORY SYSTEMS

The digestive and excretory systems consist of a large number of tissues, receptors and organs (in many ways, it makes sense to see digestion and excretion as two parts of one system). The limbic system in the brain is believed to co-ordinate appetite for food and drink. Hormones are part of the process controlling hunger and thirst. Simply thinking about food can make us hungry. It can even make some of the physical structures involved in digestion start working, long before food itself has appeared. The classic studies of dogs by Russian scientist Ivan Pavlov into the phenomenon of conditioning showed that salivation can occur when a special 'reminder' of food is introduced to an animal, even when no food is present. Think about biting into a lemon, and you may find that you suddenly start to salivate a little more.

The smell of food can make us hungry, because the nose too is part of the appetitive system. The taste buds in the tongue are involved, the salivary glands in the mouth, the throat, the stomach, the pancreas, the gall bladder, the intestines, right through to the anus. In different degrees, the actions of each may be affected by the thoughts and feelings of an individual, and illness or disease which affects any of them can also be exacerbated by worry and anxiety. When people are depressed, they often report a dulling of taste sensation, so that food loses some of its appeal. When people are very anxious they may lose their appetite, or conversely they might eat more. Stress may cause indigestion and ulcers in the stomach (small inflamed 'holes' in the stomach lining). Both diarrhoea and constipation can result from stress.

The mind is involved in almost all aspects of the digestive and excretory systems, from the choice of foodstuffs right through to toilet habits. Health psychologists have tended to concentrate on disorders of the appetite, such as anorexia nervosa and bulimia. Some work has been focused around 'fussy eating' in both children and adults. All of these areas of investigation, some of which will be explored in more depth in subsequent chapters, show the relationships between somatic systems and personality, cognition and emotion.

Furthermore, food preference is controlled by cultural mechanisms, not simply biological drives. Health psychologists need always to be aware of the cultural influences on behaviour. Different people eat different things, and this depends on their income, socio-economic status and values. There are people in England who find the prospect of eating snails and almost-raw meat truly disgusting, and there are people in France who would be equally appalled at the extent to which the English cook their beef and who find battered, fried fish seasoned with vinegar most distasteful. The difficulty is that many of the distinctions people make between good food and bad food are arbitrary. If a health psychologist (or a dietician) is helping a person to eat a 'good' diet, they might face some rather illogical principles. Many people who eat mushrooms find blue cheeses repulsive. This is despite the fact that blue cheeses are blue because they contain a fungus, and mushrooms are fungi. Arguing this point with a person who likes one but not the other is not likely to achieve anything. Food can be a very personal matter, an idiosyncratic matter, influenced by upbringing but also by some biological factors. Some people hate green vegetables. They find the taste offputting. There is now evidence that the reason for this might be genetic. Some people have a gene that allows them to taste a chemical (phenylthiocarbamide), present in green vegetables amongst other things, which is actually unpleasantly bitter (Hamer and Copeland, 2000). Those people who like green vegetables do so, perhaps, because they lack this gene, and so cannot taste something that those with the gene can. Telling people that green vegetables are good for them will not necessarily encourage them to eat them if they truly cannot bear the taste.

THE NERVOUS SYSTEM

This is arguably the most complicated system in the body. It contains the brain, which alone is made up of billions of cells with billions of connections (synapses). It is responsible for, amongst other things, the co-ordination of all of the other systems, making it the control centre. Basically, the nervous system divides into two subsystems, the central (CNS) and the peripheral (PNS). The PNS is divided into two subsystems, the somatic nervous system and the autonomic nervous system Confusingly, the autonomic nervous system is further divided into the sympathetic and parasympathetic systems!

The CNS consists of the brain and the spinal cord, both of which are massively involved in the workings of the body. The spinal cord is the structure which enables communication with the body parts below the head. Clinical psychologists, in particular, spend a lot of their time working with patients who have, either because of trauma or surgery, suffered damage to the CNS. Strokes and physical accidents are common causes of change of mood, behaviour and everyday abilities such as speech.

The PNS is made up of nerve cells and nerve bundles outside of the CNS. As stated earlier, it divides into the somatic nervous system and the autonomic nervous system. The somatic nervous system is the mode of transport of 'messages' from the CNS to the muscles and glands, and from the sense organs to the CNS. When you touch something, the signals relating to that experience reach the brain via the somatic nervous system. Select a body part – your eyes, arm, fingers, whatever – and move it, any way that you choose. The brain enables you to do this, and uses the somatic nervous system to send the right messages to your muscles to make it happen. The autonomic nervous system includes the nerve cells responsible for controlling the beating of the heart and the action of the intestines. Let us reflect on this for a moment; the heart is part of the cardiovascular system, and the intestines are part of the digestive/excretory system. Both are activated by the autonomic nervous system, which is part of the peripheral nervous system. Again, we must consider the meaningfulness of the concept of a 'system', and how closely they work together and overlap to create a functioning body.

So, we now need to turn to the two divisions of the autonomic nervous system: the sympathetic nervous system and the parasympathetic nervous system. In our world, we need people to build houses and office blocks, but we also need people to knock them down. We need a train to take us to work, and we need another to take us home again. The sympathetic and parasympathetic systems act together like this. What one system sets up, the other breaks down. The sympathetic system prepares us to face danger, either by standing up to it, or by running away (the 'fight or flight' response). It makes our heart beat more quickly and makes us breathe more heavily. It may slow down the activity of the digestive system. (When you are running for your life away from a predator it does not make sense for your body to be using up valuable energy digesting your recent sandwich.) Conversely, the parasympathetic nervous system slows down the heart rate and increases digestive activity. (Once you have got safely away from the predator, you need to calm down, rest, and allow your body to regain strength by turning the sandwich into energy.) However, it is important to realise that this does not mean that the two systems work in alternation, one-on/one-off, and then vice versa. In fact, both are working to some extent all of the time. The temporary, relative power of one over the other is what makes things happen in a particular way. In a sense, the systems constantly work together, but are also constantly in opposition. Sometimes, however, they simply co-operate to produce one ultimate effect. For example, in males, the parasympathetic system is responsible for erection of the penis, whereas the sympathetic system co-ordinates ejaculation.

The sympathetic nervous system, as has been said, is responsible for the fight-or-flight response. It is actually the basis for the stress response. Cannon (1927) described the reactions of the body to danger, suggesting why these have evolved. The blood pressure and heart rate increase, and the person sweats. The digestive system partly shuts down. Today, very few people are likely to be chased by a tiger whilst engaging in their daily activities. Current dangers are more subtle; divorce, redundancy, unemployment, petty crime, debt, sexual dysfunction, nuisance neighbours, legal disputes. These are the things that people fear today, and these are the things that cause anxiety and stress. The bodily signs of stress include increased blood pressure, increased heart rate, digestive problems, and so on. This is the irony of the stress response; it is a necessary, acute reaction to a potentially harmful situation, but chronically it can be fatal. Later in this book we will encounter more about stress and how people react to it.

THE RESPIRATORY SYSTEM

The respiratory system is the name for the apparatus involved in breathing, including the mouth, nose, trachea (windpipe), lungs and various muscles which help to force air in and out of the body. It is our way of absorbing oxygen, without which we would asphyxiate within minutes. The respiratory system feeds oxygen into the cardiovascular system. The cardiovascular system then pumps the oxygen, attached to a protein in the blood (haemoglobin), around the body, in order to 'nourish' tissues and organs. We need oxygen in the blood to survive. However, if the balance of oxygen in the blood alters, there can be drastic consequences. In the very short term, oxygen deprivation causes the body to shut down in order to preserve what little oxygen it still has; we faint. After only a few minutes, brain cells starved of oxgyen begin to die, resulting in permanent damage and, potentially, loss of function. This is one reason why, when people stop breathing, it is important to restart the respiratory processes immediately. Similarly, during parturition (birth), it is essential that the newborn begins breathing normally very quickly once exposed to the air, otherwise lifelong brain damage may result. Just as people often say, too much of a good thing can also be a very bad thing. We can be fatally poisoned by higher-than-normal concentrations of oxygen. Too high a proportion of oxygen in air, compared with the other gases present such as nitrogen, and we also permanently destroy or injure neurons. (Interestingly, we faint when we are exposed to too much oxygen too.)

So, any upsetting of the homeostatic mechanism carefully regulating breathing will result in serious damage. People who breathe too much or too little will soon feel the effects of this. Unlike most aspects of the cardiovascular system, the respiratory system can *easily* be controlled consciously. We do not have to think about breathing in order to breathe, but the moment we choose to think about breathing we assume control over it. If we want to, we can usually breathe faster or more slowly, or not at all for a while (useful when swimming, obviously). When people are anxious, they breathe differently from their normal pattern. Panic attacks often involve hyperventilation (breathing too much, too quickly), which in turn can create further panic. When people start noticing their breathing pattern, they upset its unconscious control mechanism, and, like the heart rate, concentrating on it can affect how it works.

Of course, the breathing pattern can be altered by things outside of our control. We do not breathe normally when the environment is filled with smoke, or car exhaust fumes and so on. Equally, asthma is a condition where breathing can be severely restricted despite the person's efforts to bring their breathing under control. What is of interest here is that many doctors believe that the anxiety caused by the breathing difficulties associated with an asthmatic attack may serve to create further breathing problems. Thus, the person is caught in a cycle of strained breathing causing anxiety causing strained breathing and so on. Not only can a bout of asthma be brought on by anxiety, but the psychological component in this illness was clearly demonstrated by a number of studies including Butler and Steptoe (1986) who gave asthmatic participants a harmless (placebo) solution to inhale. Some were told that this was an irritant, and they developed symptoms of asthma accordingly, whereas those who were not told this did not. Furthermore, if people were given a pretend asthma drug followed by the pretend irritant, there were fewer symptoms of asthma recorded.

THE CARDIOVASCULAR SYSTEM

The cardiovascular system includes the heart itself, and the veins, arteries, venules, capillaries and other vessels which feed into and out of it. It is essentially the means of transport of oxygen from the respiratory system, and also of nutrients, waste products and toxins. The digestive system provides nutrients which end up in the blood and are taken to tissues to assist in their upkeep. Their metabolic processes generate waste products (which are often toxins) which are then transported, again by the blood, to the excretory system. (The respiratory system also serves as an excretory mechanism, getting rid of poisons like carbon dioxide by means of exhalation.) Health psychologists tend to be most interested in the cardiovascular system in two ways. They concentrate on the heart rate and the blood pressure. Both of these, if anything other than normal, can create serious challenges to health, and, indeed, cognitive functioning. An unhealthy or unfit person tends to have a much higher heart rate, and may have abnormal blood pressure. Cholesterol levels can be dangerously high in a person who eats certain foods, which is an example of how culture and lifestyle impact upon the health state of a person. Health psychologists must take all of these factors into account. When we are anxious or stressed, the cardiovascular system is put under additional strain. This is directly linked to mortality. There are some biologists who believe that the number of heartbeats an animal has is limited in some way, and that the reason that tortoises live for a long time is that they have very slow heartbeats, whereas mice have a short lifespan because their hearts beat so quickly. If there is some truth in this, then anything which slows down the human heart rate (such as relaxation and general fitness) must be good for us.

BIOLOGICAL RHYTHMS

Of late, an increasing amount of research has been directed at the topic of circadian (daily) and other rhythms ('body-clock' timing mechanisms). There is no doubt that the body works on sleep–wake cycles, for instance. Jet-lag demonstrates what happens when the cycle is disrupted. The temperature of the body fluctuates within a day, too. Human beings are creatures of habit and routine, at least some of the time. These circadian rhythms may provide some of the structure for that routine. There are potentially serious consequences for health if a person works a range of shifts and so rarely sleeps during the same hours more than a few days in succession.

A part of the brain has been identified which might be the body's timing mechanism: the suprachiasmatic nucleus. It is part of the hypothalamus, in the forebrain. The SCN, as it is often called, produces its own rhythms. It uses light to help set the rhythm, which can mean that people who are neurally blind (i.e. they might have no eyes or retina or optic nerve) work to different daily rhythms from people with sight. The SCN regulates the production of a hormone called melatonin from the pineal gland. When you produce more melatonin, you feel like sleeping.

The menstrual cycle is governed by a 28-day timer in most women. Of course, one of the most common causes of menstrual irregularity is stress. When women are anxious, their periods may be late, lighter or heavier than usual, or they may miss a period altogether. So, stress may cause a missed period. The missed period causes further stress, perhaps because the woman may be concerned that she is pregnant. This additional stress may be implicated in even more menstrual dysfunction.

There is also some evidence that longer term, external rhythms can be related to depression. People with Seasonal Affective Disorder (SAD) respond to the seasonal changes in light availability by feeling happier during summer and becoming depressed in the winter (in areas of the earth where the amount of sunlight differs seasonally). Furthermore, the circadian rhythms of people who are depressed differ from those of people with SAD, and both differ from those of people who have neither (Teicher *et al*, 1997).

Research into bodily rhythms is still relatively new. However, it is becoming clear that there are distinct rhythms, natural ebbs and flows, if you like. Since most of these seem to be exerting some kind of psychological effect, such as in pre-menstrual syndrome or in the case of SAD, psychologists need to be aware of these, especially when studying individuals. We have long known that, for the purposes of experimental studies, all groups in our research designs need to be tested at the same time of day, in similar conditions and so on. When observing more complicated behaviours, such as smoking or drinking, diaries are a useful research tool, since they allow us to pinpoint daily weaknesses in willpower, or times of the month when a person might be best equipped, psychologically, to give up smoking or to take up exercise.

THE STRESS RESPONSE

Health psychologists have a particular interest in responses to stress. As has been seen repeatedly in this chapter, disorders in systems can generate stress, and stress can create disorders in systems. This is why health psychology often boils down to a study of stress. Stress will be dealt with separately elsewhere in this book, but it is appropriate to outline the biological mechanisms supporting the stress response here.

Stress is the natural response to a danger or concern that an organism faces. It prepares the organism for potential trouble. As was mentioned earlier, stress is what happens to a person when they are in 'fight-or-flight' response mode. When danger is faced, or anticipated, the following things happen.

- Heart rate changes, and strength of heartbeat changes. Usually, both increase, but the opposite may happen. In the most common situation, what happens is that the heart rate and so on change to allow more blood to be pumped around the body quickly. What the person perceives is a fast pulse, and, commonly, palpitations. Palpitations are a sign of stress.
- Blood pressure increases. Whilst it is usual for people not to notice blood pressure changes directly (although some people do say that they can feel it, especially after a heavy meal), they tend to notice the consequences of blood pressure increases such as headaches. It is hardly surprising, then, that headaches are a classic symptom of stress.
- Blood vessels in skin alter in girth. Usually, they constrict, but they may dilate. Constriction serves the purpose of directing blood towards the muscles and organs which require it as a priority. As a result, people may go much paler than they usually are. In some cases, they become flushed and more pink. Black people undergo exactly the same changes, but they are generally less noticeable than in white people.

- Muscles become prepared for action by increased blood flow to them. Stressed people are said to be 'tense', and may require methods such as massage to loosen up the muscles which the body has put into a state of preparation for activity, in anticipation of trouble.
- Sweat glands begin to work harder. This cools the body down to prevent overheating. However, the stressed person (and their friends and family) may notice that they have more bodily odour than previously. The person may notice that deodorants don't seem to work as well for them as they used to. They may be noticeably wet on the brow, or under the arms or on the back.
- Lungs can take in more air because the air passages open up. Stressed people may breathe unevenly, perhaps taking in deeper breaths than might seem necessary. Frequency of sighing might be increased. As a result of increased activity, the lungs might become sensitive, causing them to shut off; asthma is something that is more likely to be found in people who are anxious, and stressed.
- Pupils of the eyes dilate. This allows more light to be let in, thus giving the eyes a better chance of picking out danger. However, to other people, it may look strange. The stare of a stressed person can be quite different from that of a relaxed one.
- Salivation is temporarily turned off. Generally, the body does not need saliva during a dangerous situation. The body's energy is better used on other things. Therefore, the mouth becomes dry. Dryness of the mouth is another sign of stress.
- Digestive processes are altered. Depending on the nature of the situation, food in the stomach may need to be held there until later, or it may need to be digested quickly. In the former case, it is kept in the stomach longer than usual, and in the latter case increased secretions of gastric acids can lead to damage to the stomach itself. It is not unusual for people with chronic stress problems to develop stomach ulcers.
- Intestinal activity is changed. Again, the situation may call for a suspension of bowel activity, or it might call for increased attention to it. If the dangerous situation is pre-empted, it makes sense for the body to get rid of waste. Running away from a predator is easier if you are a few ounces lighter. Thus diarrhoea can occur. However, if the danger is immediate, the system is designed to stop bowel activity, thus saving energy for fight or flight. As a consequence, constipation occurs. Irregularities in the function of the bowel are another classic symptom of stress.

Given what happens to a stressed body, it is easy to see how long-term bouts of stress can place considerable strain upon the biological systems and often damage them irreparably. Stress is a major source of health problems in many countries, as will be seen elsewhere in this book.

Interestingly, small amounts of stress might be good for a person, since they can be viewed as a form of 'exercise' of the cardiovascular and respiratory systems. Moderate exercise is beneficial precisely because it makes us breathe more quickly and more deeply, and it causes the blood pressure to temporarily rise, the heart rate to increase, and so on. Therefore, occasional stress can be a form of moderate exercise. Positive stress is often termed **eustress**.

PSYCHONEUROIMMUNOLOGY

This is a relatively new field of psychological medicine. It has caught the imagination of many health psychologists because it involves a strong and explicit recognition of the relationship between mind and body. The immune system itself is vital in the upkeep of the human body. It is responsible for defending the body against the onslaught of bacteria and viruses, and is also implicated in diseases such as cancer. There is now evidence that the functioning of the immune system (immunocompetence) can be affected by the workings of the mind.

It is probably a mistake to think that diseases can be defeated simply by the 'power of the mind', 'mind over matter', or 'positive thinking'. It is no more sensible than the view that a person can die because they 'lose the will to live' or 'give up the ghost'. However, attitude can have *some* effect on the course of an illness, and might even tip the balance in some people. Basically, the key link is between stress and the immune response. Evidence exists to suggest that the immune system works less well when a person is undergoing stress. Anything that detrimentally affects the immune system certainly weakens the organism.

Cohen *et al* (1993) studied the effects of infection by the common cold virus comparing people who reported having had a number of significantly stressful life events with those who had not. Common-sense notions that when bad things happen to people it toughens them up were not supported. It weakens them, if anything. After infection with the virus under controlled conditions, those people who had reported more stressful events in the previous year had higher temperatures than those who had lived less stressful lives of late. They also reported more nasal mucus, one of the characteristic signs of having a cold, as the reader will be aware. These were not purely psychogenic symptoms. A placebo group of people who were not subjected to the cold virus (but who *thought* that they *might* have been) did not develop these symptoms, even if they were people who had reported high levels of stress in the 12 months prior to the study. So, it seems that if a person becomes ill, stressful events really can make them more ill.

Additionally, it is not only minor illnesses such as the common cold where stress-related deficits in the immune system might create challenges to the organism. There is a considerable body of work looking at stress and immunity in relation to cancer, one of the world's most common causes of death. Visintainer *et al* (1982) injected rats with cancerous cells and then electrically shocked them to create stress. The rats were either able to escape the shocks or they were not. They found that tumours grew more readily in those rats subjected to inescapable shocks. The unavoidable trauma clearly affected the animals' resistance to the injected cells. Sklar and Anisman (1981) demonstrated a link between contracting cancer and self-reports of stress. Those people with cancer had been significantly stressed prior to their symptoms, which leads some to suggest that the immune system was impaired because of stress, which then allowed cancerous cells to develop unchecked. However, studies of this kind are difficult to interpret since people with cancer may report greater stresses prior to diagnosis because they are under such stress at the time of filling in the questionnaire. When one wears sunglasses all day it is easy to forget what the world looks like without them. Similarly, the diagnosis of cancer is not the point at which it begins. Most of the participants in such a study would have had some biological evidence of cancer prior to diagnosis, and may have been worried about unusual symptoms for some time before consulting a doctor. Thus, the cancer itself may have created stress prior to it being formally detected.

Stress can affect the functioning of the immune system in two ways, physiologically, through chemical effects, and behaviourally, through people's responses to stress which can then damage the body further. Not only does stress cause chemicals to be released which can affect immunocompetence, but also a person who is stressed is more likely to smoke, drink alcohol, take other drugs, and eat poorly, all of which have an impact on immunocompetence.

Stress, physiology and immune dysfunction

When a person is stressed, their body generates more cortisol and catecholamines, as explained earlier. It is thought that higher levels of these substances can suppress the activity of the immune system. Whilst viruses, poisons and so on cause many illnesses, exposure to a virus or toxin does not always mean that the illness can take hold. The immune system, ideally, fights the incoming virus and destroys it or renders it incapable, or it neutralises or catabolises (breaks down) the toxin in some way. When the person is stressed, the immune system is less able to do its job. This means that they are more likely to become ill, but also more likely to remain ill for longer and have worse symptoms.

The details of how, chemically and otherwise, the immune system is affected by stress will not be dealt with in this book because this is not a book on psychoneuroimmunology. Suffice it to say that cortisol and the catecholamines prepare the body for action, and opiates (the body's natural painkillers) are produced, which also might have an immunosuppressive effect (O'Leary, 1990).

Behavioural causes of immune dysfunction

Not all immune system problems are caused by stressors. Common drugs, such as alcohol, can also have an effect. Higher doses of alcohol can cause reproductive 'sluggishness' of lymphocytes, the white blood cells which create antigens which, in turn, deal with foreign bodies in the blood (Johnson *et al*, 1981). Smoking may also be implicated in immune system dysfunction. Aside from any direct effects on the immune system, smoking can have an effect on the respiratory tract, meaning that the filtering processes in the lungs are less efficient. Since the lungs are a primary filter for airborne toxins entering the body, damaging the lungs in any way could give the immune system additional work to do.

Therefore, we can see again that aspects of behaviour impact indirectly on health status, in this case by exerting an influence on the efficiency of the immune system. People choose to smoke and drink alcohol, and this choice has its price for health in obvious and much less obvious ways.

Types of stress

However, we must draw a distinction between chronic and acute stress. There is some evidence that chronic stressors might (sometimes) actually serve to enhance immune function rather than suppress it. If you are stressed for a long time, you might adjust to it. Getting used to stress, so that it becomes a way of life, may alter your biological baselines. If all of your systems adjust, then chronic stress may cease to have the characteristic effects of stress (Monjan, 1981). However, chronic stress is a serious problem in its own right, which will be discussed in Chapter 5.

CONCLUDING REMARKS

This chapter has demonstrated that the mind and the body are clearly linked systems. They work together, but changes in the way that the body works can create some subtle and some much more dramatic changes in the way that the organism or person behaves. There are many ways in which the body can influence the mind, because there are a number of interwoven systems which can go wrong, having consequences for the person. In many cases, bodily dysfunction can lead to behavioural dysfunction which in turn can lead to greater bodily dysfunction. Thus cycles of damage can occur which are difficult to break. Many substances and processes can affect the body in two ways: either by their surfeit or by their surplus. For these substances, moderation appears to be the path the body naturally takes. This balance biologists refer to as homeostasis. Table 2.1 summarises a selection of these.

Table 2.1 Balances in the body

Consequences of deficit	Substance/process/action	Consequences of surfeit
Cell death	Oxygen	Cell death
Death	Water	Heart failure
Deficiency diseases, death	Food	Obesity, which if unrestrained will lead to heart disease and death
Atrophy of the muscles, cardiovascular disease, possible fatality	Exercise	Strain on cardiovascular system, possible fatality
Various diseases and eventually death	Vitamins	Various diseases and eventually death
Even teetotallers may take in alcohol in small amounts in foods like fruits and bread. There is evidence that in small amounts alcohol may benefit health (Jackson *et al*, 1991)	Alcohol	Alcoholism, organ damage, Korsakoff's Syndrome, death
Hypotension is associated with kidney failure and is a common symptom of drug overdose	Blood Pressure	Chronic hypertension is associated with strokes and myocardial infarction
Bradychardia (slow heart rate) is often a sign of heart disease	Heart Rate	Tachycardia (fast heart rate) is often a sign of heart disease
Hypothyroidism	Thyroxine	Hyperthyroidism
Without saturated fat, the body cannot conduct normal metabolic processes	Saturated Fat	Atherosclerosis, arteriosclerosis, heart disease, death
Depression	Serotonin	Mania
Parkinson's disease	Dopamine	Schizophrenia

Study questions

1. Looking at each of the systems outlined in this chapter in turn, identify what people commonly feel when they experience problems with their functioning. What are the psychosocial consequences of a dysfunction of each?

2. How might problems with the endocrine, digestive/excretory, nervous, respiratory and cardiovascular systems exert an influence on normal sexual functioning?

FURTHER READING

Kalat, J.W. (1998): *Biological Psychology, Sixth Edition*. Pacific Grove, CA: Brooks/Cole. A standard textbook used by many undergraduates, giving a good overview of the body's functions and their interrelationship with the mind.

Lovallo, W.R. (1997): *Stress and Health: Biological and Psychological Interactions*. London: Sage. A book dealing with the biological and psychological nature of the stress response and its impact on health.

3 Perceptions, Beliefs and Cognitions

INTRODUCTION

What people think about their health, and how they perceive illness (both generally and their own), is fundamental to health psychology. Different writers and researchers on the subject divide up this area in a number of ways, but in many respects the distinctions are artificial. If someone thinks something, then they tend to believe it. If they perceive something a certain way, they are likely to think along the lines of that perception, and have faith in their perception. If they believe something, their thoughts will often spring from their beliefs. Perceptions, beliefs and cognitions may all lead to one thing: behaviour. Therefore, health behaviours (things people do which may enhance or injure their health), need to be understood at the level of their under-pinnings. If we know why people do something, we can work with them to alter it.

LAY MODELS

A useful starting point is the models of health and illness that people construct for themselves, often referred to as **naïve** or **common-sense** models. We do not need to say a great deal about these, partly because they often surface naturally when we use the psychologists' models, but we need to be aware that people can create fairly complicated systems of belief surrounding their health, but they often lack the training or knowledge to test out those beliefs in the way that a health researcher could. Consequently, their naïve beliefs often go unchecked and unopposed. For example, a person might refuse to stop smoking because, in their experience, no-one ever seemed to die of smoking, despite what the 'experts' say. If they have never known a person to die of lung cancer who smoked, but perhaps knew a non-smoker who did develop the disease, and had a number of long-living family members and friends who were heavy smokers, then they develop a model that fits the evidence of their senses. Of course, the fact of the matter is that basing a theory on a handful of examples when the 'experts' have based theirs on, literally, tens or hundreds of thousands is a mistaken strategy. But for that person, a model has been generated which may take some shaking before it is adapted or replaced by the more appropriate one. For instance, research by Cornwell (1984) showed that 92% of the working-class people interviewed in East London did not believe that smoking caused cancer. Most put forward that it might trigger off a cancer which already existed, but it would not create a new one. Providing those people with evidence that they will accept may prove a mammoth task.

It is not uncommon for people to believe that it is possible to catch a cold from exposure to cold air, and more specifically, a drenching in cold water (Helman, 1995). Most of us will have witnessed scenes in movies and soap operas where a character accidentally gets very wet and then develops a very bad cold. Whilst it is true that a shock to the system such as being immersed in water might easily temporarily affect the functioning of the immune system, it is not possible to catch a cold without being exposed to the relevant virus, something almost exclusively done by someone who is infected breathing, coughing, sneezing or spitting onto our faces. Despite this, parents are sometimes heard telling their children to come inside out of the rain to stop them catching a cold.

These lay notions of health can affect quite significantly the extent to which people will comply with advice given to them by a doctor. If you do not believe that smoking is unhealthy for you, you will not readily take a doctor's advice to desist from smoking, especially since you might feel that smoking does you some good because it helps to calm your nerves. Another example of a potentially damaging lay belief is that provided by Mulatu (1999), who studied Ethiopian attitudes towards both mental and physical illness. Four factors explained the variance in beliefs about the causes of illness; psychosocial stressors, supernature, physical defects and socio-environmental deprivation. Whilst three of these are well known to health psychologists as genuine causes of ill health, supernatural causes have not been considered. Had health psychology originated in Africa instead of in North America and Europe, supernature might have attracted more attention. The difficulty arises in that mental illness in particular is seen as having some supernatural cause, perhaps as a form of vengeance by spirits for something that the person has done wrong. Therefore, treatments for mental illness offered by doctors might not satisfy the patient nor their family unless the supernatural element is included. In addition, there is a belief that contagion is possible in such cases, which may mean that a person is more isolated than they might be. Since mental illness is often something which can be handled well with social support, the belief in Ethiopia that people who are mentally ill might be contagious could mean that they are denied necessary social support.

THE HEALTH BELIEF MODEL (HBM)

Possibly the most important body of work in this area, certainly historically, is the study around the Health Belief Model (see Fig. 3.1). This dates back to Rosenstock (1966), and has been frequently used as a framework for understanding health beliefs since then. Because the model has been adapted and modified a number of times, it is difficult to present a single version of it. In your reading you will find many different descriptions of what the authors call the HBM. In essence, however, they are very similar and are mostly based around six themes. At times, some of these are conjoined; severity and susceptibility have often been seen as one theme of health 'threat', but as Sheeran and Abraham (1995) point out, they are best looked at separately. So, do not be perturbed when you read about versions of this model that do not match exactly the one outlined below. Alternative models are all based around the same fundamental concepts. It does not perhaps help that it is conventional to speak of *the* HBM, as if there were only one, which was always the same.

To predict the likelihood that a person will engage in a particular health behaviour in response to a specific health threat (like a potential illness or disease), the HBM requires that we consider what the person *perceives* as the **costs** and **benefits** of engaging in the health behaviour (sometimes expanded to **barriers** and **benefits**), what they *perceive* as the **severity** of the threat, what they *perceive* as their personal **susceptibility** to the threat, and any **cues to action** that exist or occur, which can come from inside the individual or outside of them. A cue to action is something that acts as a prompt to the person to do something to protect their health. It might be a symptom or sign in their body, or it might come in the form of advice from a doctor or a friend. Note that perceptions are all important. The real threat a person faces does not matter at all. People act only on perceived threats. (Of course, if a person happens to know the facts and statistics about a disease, then their perceived threat might match very closely the actual threat.) There is one other principal issue to be considered, which was included in later formulations of the model (Becker *et al*, 1977). This is **health motivation**. This is a way of describing a

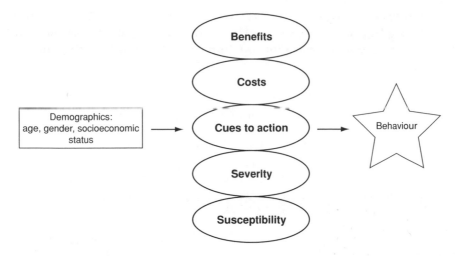

Fig. 3.1 The early Health Belief Model

person's interest in health matters, and the extent to which they are generally motivated to act on the issue of health.

We can now look at how each of these things can be turned into real thoughts and feelings concerning health. If we take a woman in her twenties who intends losing weight, these are the things she might think and the relevant circumstances surrounding her actions.

Case in Point: Helen

Costs
'Diet food and health food can be quite expensive.' 'Shopping with a diet in mind can be stressful and time-consuming.' 'I will not be able to eat what I like and treat myself to food.' 'I will have to buy a new wardrobe of clothes which will cost a fortune.' 'I will get irritable and anxious unless I eat what I like when I like.'

Benefits
'I will be happier and healthier.' 'I will be more attractive to some people.' 'I will be much less likely to develop a wide range of diseases.' 'I will be able to exercise more freely.' 'I will feel sad less often, because eating too much and being fat makes me sad sometimes.'

Health motivation
'I care about my health, and want to be healthy.' 'I find the human body quite interesting, and will often read the health sections of magazines.'

Susceptibility
'Being fat can make you diabetic, and my mother is a big woman who is diabetic.' 'Being fat can make you die early, and longevity is not a characteristic of my family.' 'My father has angina, and so there's some evidence of heart disease in the family.' 'Two of my uncles died of strokes.' 'Overall, I would say that I'm pretty much at risk if I stay this size.'

Severity
'Diabetes is a serious illness and can be fatal. Heart disease is too.' 'Dying younger than average is not a pleasant thought.'

Cues to action
'I notice some people looking at me and I know that they are probably thinking about my size.' 'I sometimes get the feeling that people do not find me attractive.' 'I cannot find clothes to fit me easily.' 'I get out of breath quickly and cannot run properly.' 'I get all sorts of aches and pains which I reckon are because my body is carrying excess weight.' 'The last time I visited the doctor she checked my blood pressure and it was too high. She advised me to lose weight.'

The model also allows for demographic variables and psychological characteristics which might affect health beliefs which in turn then feed into the model to enable a prediction of the likelihood of action. After all, some of the beliefs a person holds do not simply come from themselves, but from their culture, society, and so on. Some ideas and values do stem from a basic make-up of the person: what kind of personality they have. Both 'influences' are important in shaping beliefs.

Before we make our prediction that this person will engage in the health behaviour in question, that is dieting, we should, therefore, consider these two groups of factors.

Demographic variables
This person is a young female. Research shows that young women are particularly likely to engage in dieting behaviour.

Psychological characteristics
Helen is markedly the most overweight of her social group, and she tends to be susceptible to peer pressure. She has a good selection of supportive friends. She has an internal locus of control (believing that she exerts most influence over her own life), and she tends to use problem-focused, rather than emotion-focused, coping. Therefore, she prefers to work things out rather than focus on her feelings.

Putting this together, we can start to create a picture of the future for this person. Using statistical techniques which will not be detailed here, it becomes possible to judge whether she will actually take on the challenge of dieting to lose weight. You can see that she clearly does perceive herself to be susceptible to weight-related health threats, she does see the consequences of obesity as serious, she is the right type of person in the right social circumstances to diet, she is motivated towards health issues, and the cues to action are strong. Helen has a good chance of succeeding in dieting. We must weigh this up against the costs of dieting which she has outlined. Of course, this is where we face difficulties. How exactly can we begin to determine if those costs to her outweigh the other factors? The thoughts she has expressed do not come with values attached to them. This is where careful scaling of items in the questionnaire can be of use (see Chapter 8 on psychometric testing). By looking at how much this person agrees or disagrees with various statements it becomes possible to compare the 'fors and againsts' in a numerical fashion. Some authors suggest that the benefits and barriers should be calculated as a pair or one subtracted from the other (Becker and Maiman, 1975). This aside, the reader should be able to see that the HBM covers most, if not all, of the factors which, on the face of it, should be relevant in determining if a person engages in a particular behaviour. Of course, the case above is artificial, since it concerns one individual, and most research into the HBM is conducted on groups, to discover which factors from those above are most important for most people, most of the time. One more point must be considered. Although we can make predictions about Helen's success in dieting, we have to reconsider all of the variables once she has begun to do so. Maintenance of a health behaviour is quite different from the initiation of it. Just because she begins losing weight does not mean that she will reach her target weight and remain at that level for the rest of her life.

We now can turn to a real piece of research using the HBM, this time investigating adolescent condom use in Scotland, as reported by Sheeran and Abraham (1995). Two sets of adolescents were identified, those at 16 and those at 18 years of age. An HBM-based questionnaire was sent out, yielding 690 returns, and it was sent out again one year later. Pairing up the questionnaires, the researchers ended up with 333 responses which they could use. Questions included those about intended condom use. Their results were not encouraging, in that HBM components did not predict condom use (and thus HIV-preventative behaviour). They suggest that it might be the case that safer-sex health beliefs are essentially in place for all participants, but that other factors lead to actual health behaviour. However, the results were complicated by a gender difference in the relationship between intention and behaviour. For males, there was a small but significant relationship between the two, but for women there was not. The authors argue that this might reflect the lack of choice women may feel that they have in sexual relationships. If a man chooses to wear a condom he might find it easy to translate this choice into action, whereas, prior to the creation of the female condom, a woman has to rely on a man to use this contraceptive device. This shows that the HBM, whilst a good starting point for health psychologists, misses out on a great many other factors which determine behaviour. For this reason, other models have since taken precedence.

THE PROTECTION MOTIVATION THEORY (PMT)

A further development from the HBM is the Protection Motivation Theory (PMT) (Rogers, 1975; 1983). This is illustrated in Fig. 3.2. Again, like the HBM, there are a number of versions of the model in existence. They posit the suggestion that there are a set of predictors of people's *intentions* to behave in a certain way, which lead directly to their actual behaviour. It gets its name from the notion that people are motivated to protect themselves by acting to preserve health. They appraise both the threat they face, and their own coping mechanisms and skill. They develop an intention to perform (or to maintain) either a behaviour which is going to protect their health (protection motivation, or adaptive response) or even damage it (a maladaptive response). A maladaptive coping response might be smoking more cigarettes or eating more chocolate after being told you have signs of heart disease, or denying the problem entirely and dismissing the doctors' advice.

So, in assessing the threat that they face, people take into account three factors, **fear, perceived severity** of the illness and **perceived vulnerability** to it. (This will be looking familiar to the reader by now.) In assessing their coping, people consider **self-efficacy** and the **response efficacy**. The first of these is their beliefs about their ability to perform the desired, adaptive response. The

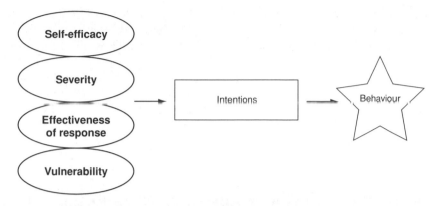

Fig. 3.2 A schematic representation of Protection Motivation Theory

response efficacy is essentially their beliefs about how likely it is that the behaviour they are aiming for will actually help them by reducing a health threat. In both stages, costs and benefits/advantages and disadvantages of the aimed-for behaviour and the damaging behaviour are taken into account.

Kanvil and Umeh (2000) looked at both the HBM and PMT in understanding cigarette use and the threats posed by lung cancer. Questionnaires were completed by 275 undergraduate students. The researchers aimed to predict intentions to smoke from the some features of the two models, including fear and perceived vulnerability. Using a statistical technique called multiple regression, they attempted to explain motivation to smoke using scores on other factors, such as components of the models, age and gender. Regression analysis yields a number which can be converted into a percentage, and this is the proportion of scores in one variable which can be predicted using one or more other factors. For example, we might say that we can predict height from weight, but only within certain limits. Those limits are given as a percentage of variance, such as 50%. This means that 50% of the height scores are explained by other things, not weight. So, back to Kanvil and Umeh (2000). They found that only 3% of motivation to smoke could be predicted using health cognition factors! This means that 97% of the scores have nothing to do with fear, or perceived threat or perceived vulnerability or perceived barriers to quitting. However, the prediction improved to 70% when past behaviour was included in the regression model. This means that most of smoking motivation can be explained now, and most of that by reference to past behaviour. This might seem common sense, to say that if a person smoked last week they will smoke this week. In a sense it is rather obvious. What is important is that neither the HBM nor the PMT actually incorporate past behaviour as an intrinsically important variable. In both, past behaviour is seen as a moderating factor, but something rather external, like social pressure.

What these researchers have shown is that the models seriously miss out on a highly predictive variable. What someone did before *does* have a profound significance for what they are likely to do next. What they also suggest is that future intentions may affect perceived risk. Therefore, a person who intends giving up smoking in a year's time may perceive their chances of developing lung cancer as lower because of it. This may in turn impact on their present behaviour. We can see, then, that our models are constantly being refined, and are still in their infancy. Furthermore, what may apply to smoking behaviour may not apply to eating, or alcohol consumption, or condom use.

THE THEORY OF PLANNED BEHAVIOUR (TPB)

Like many health psychology models, the Theory of Planned Behaviour (TPB) developed from work in social psychology, specifically the theory of reasoned action. Ajzen (1985, 1988, 1991) indicated that Perceived Behavioural Control (PBC) affects intentions, and that intentions then influence actual behaviour. PBC works in conjunction with two other factors, which are **subjective norms** and **attitudes to behaviour**. Let us consider what each of these terms might mean. PBC is the extent to which a person perceives that they are in control of their behaviour and are thus going to be able to achieve a desired health behaviour, such as eating more carbohydrate/less fat, or exercising. This is a belief based not only on intrinsic factors such as personality and ability, but extrinsic ones such as personal finances and so on. Subjective norms are beliefs about the desirability of carrying out a certain health behaviour in the society, social group and culture in which the person lives. Attitudes to behaviour are simply what they sound like. Every person will have attitudes towards performing a certain behaviour, either good or bad, and attitudes towards the end result or outcome of that behaviour. Whether or not someone genuinely intends to perform a behaviour will depend on a combination of what society tells them about that behaviour, what they feel they are capable of doing, and what their attitudes to that behaviour and the potential result of it will be. A person addicted to heroin might have strong beliefs that heroin addiction is not socially acceptable, especially if their friends and family are disapproving (subjective norms), might have a positive attitude to shrugging off the addiction and the outcome of doing so, such as becoming a normal citizen again and acquiring work (attitudes to behaviour), but they might not have much belief that they are capable of giving up the drug, especially since it is highly addictive psychologically (PBC). As a consequence, their intention to give up heroin might be low, and so they are not likely to engage in that behaviour.

An early test of the theory in health came through research conducted by Schifter and Ajzen (1985) looking at weight loss in female students. They were enrolled in the study to lose weight over a period of six weeks. At the beginning of the study their attitudes to weight loss were probed, as were their opinions about dieting norms, intentions as to losing weight, and their perceived ability to manage their weight loss. Intention to lose weight was significantly predicted by subjective norms, attitudes and perceived control. Of course, you might now wonder if these things predicted weight loss in these women. Intention to lose weight and perceived control did predict some of the actual weight loss, but not as much as the researchers might have liked. The most interesting finding, it might be argued, was that intention to lose weight predicted weight loss only in those people with higher perceived behavioural control. In other words, the women who intended to lose weight but did not think that they would manage to eat fewer calories every day for six weeks were able to lose much less weight compared with those women who had the intention *and* believed that they were capable of executing the behaviour in question. In common-sense terms, the best of intentions are not enough if a person does not really believe in themselves and their ability to carry out those intentions.

SELF-EFFICACY THEORY

A number of theorists suggest that perceived self-efficacy (a belief, naturally) is a primary determinant of health behaviour (for instance, Schwarzer, 1992). This is remarkably close to what the TPB and PMT are based on: an idea of perceived control affecting behaviour. Again, we can see that key features of one model turn up in others. Schwarzer's work is often called the Health Action Process Approach (HAPA). The emphasis on a process is highly significant; in this model the person moves from one set of plans and cognitions to another in their decision-making process, which, ideally, leads to an intention to act and then measurable behaviour. Before people can act, they have to be motivated to act. The motivation phase of this model involves the person's perceived self-efficacy (if they believe they are able to act and act well), their assessment of the health threat (how severe the threat is and how vulnerable to it they are), and their outcome expectancies (what they think will happen if they do act).

Providing that people have enough perceived self-efficacy, view the outcome of the health behaviour to be beneficial, and see the threat of the illness or disease as sufficiently strong, they will then act. In the second phase (often referred to as the volitional stage), people must think positively and constructively about the health behaviour and how to achieve it (cognitive factors which can be termed 'action plans') and they must have appropriate social support and finances and so on (situational or environmental factors). Self-efficacy permeates this volitional phase too, since action plans are bound to be based on what the person realistically thinks that they can do. There is no use setting goals which you have no confidence in yourself to achieve.

Povey *et al* (2000) investigated the TPB in dietary behaviours, but with reference to the additional factors of perceived control and self-efficacy. They asked questions about behaviour and intentions towards eating a low-fat diet and eating five portions of fruit and vegetables daily. Part of the purpose of the study was to identify whether PBC and self-efficacy are separate concepts, since some have argued that they are one and the same thing. Povey *et al* suggest that they are different, and that PBC refers to whether a person believes that they can make a difference to their own behaviour and that self-efficacy is specifically related to how difficult the person perceives the proposed health behaviour to be. They found that both factors predicted intentions to have a low-fat diet and eat fruit and vegetables, but that the stronger predictor of the two was self-efficacy. They argue that a person's intentions to perform a behaviour are affected more by how difficult they think that behaviour would be to engage in, rather than how much they think they would be in control of their behaviour. Whilst the authors use these findings to support the TPB, there is also evidence here that self-efficacy theory has its place.

Bray *et al* (2001) looked at self-efficacy in relation to attendance at exercise classes. However, they also investigated the role of what is called **proxy efficacy**. It leads on from the issue of proxy control, which is basically handing over some or all of the control over a certain issue to another person, for any number of reasons. Most democratic parliaments work this way, in that once we have elected a particular member of parliament or government, we expect them to deal with issues on our behalf. Proxy efficacy, therefore, is the extent to which we believe that a person has the skills and abilities required to assist us or carry out duties on our behalf. In the case of exercise classes, the proxy in question is the fitness instructor who leads the classes. In a study over a number of weeks, they researched 127 women who were attending fitness classes. They found that there was a small but significant relationship between proxy efficacy and self-efficacy. Therefore, the extent to which someone believes that a powerful other (the instructor) is capable and efficient relates to the extent to which they believe that they can overcome barriers to their own success in a health behaviour context. Looking at attendance, the researchers split the women into experienced exercisers and novices. Self-efficacy and proxy efficacy predicted attendance moderately in the novices, but there was no observed prediction in the experienced exercisers. What this tells us is that when people are starting to take up exercise, a good instructor can 'make or break' their success. Of course, in terms of self-efficacy theory, this study shows us that not only does self-efficacy influence health behaviours, but that proxy efficacy, where appropriate, must also be taken into account. In addition, the contribution of these factors to the performance of health behaviour depends upon the experience of the person.

SELF-REGULATORY MODEL

Leventhal *et al*'s (1980) self-regulatory model is a model of illness cognitions. Interestingly enough, Leventhal defines illness cognitions using the word 'beliefs'. In that sense, the distinctions between health beliefs and illness cognitions are a little artificial. Health beliefs are things that people think about health, and illness cognitions are things that people think about illness. Since health and illness are terms which come from the same semantic field, a study of what people believe about their health is, perhaps, complemented by what they think about illness.

Leventhal's model is essentially dynamic and compensatory in nature. When a person becomes ill they adjust themselves to the new situation, and the model describes that adjustment. This adjustment takes the form of solving a problem. Hence, you will occasionally find Leventhal's model referred to as a problem-solving approach. Like all problems or puzzles, we aim to take the information we have (referred to by cognitive psychologists as **givens**) and convert it into a solution. According to Leventhal, the givens are classifiable in five ways.

- **Identity:** This is simply the name of the disease or illness, as gained from a diagnosis from the doctor, or, perhaps, from self-diagnosis, and the symptoms. It is the label the person gives to the changed state, and a description of that state.
- **Perceived cause:** This is exactly what it sounds like. People make a more-or-less informed guess as to the reason why they are ill. It could be based on folk myth, actual medical knowledge or fantasy.
- **Time line:** This is the perceived timescale for the disease or illness. Again, based on either supposition or knowledge, the person guesses as to how long they can expect to be ill, or how long each phase of an illness might last.
- **Consequences:** This is where the person predicts the financial, emotional, physical, and other outcomes of being ill. The consequences of the illness might be perceived as being trivial or serious.
- **Control and cure:** This is a twofold belief. It concerns perceptions of the possibility that the illness can be cured or ameliorated, and perceptions of control over the illness, either by the individual themselves or by friends, medical professionals, and any other powerful others.

The self-regulatory model is divided into three stages (**interpretation, coping** and **appraisal**), and the dimensions of cognitions above apply to the first stage, **interpretation** of the illness. They are the ways in which people think about their illness which create a representation of that illness. You cannot begin to do something about being ill unless you get to grips with the illness itself and what it seems to involve. This is your interpretation of it. Your interpretation of the illness involves also an **emotional response**, which might feed back into your interpretation. If you have thought long and hard about your illness, and you have set up a cognitive framework for understanding it, you will also have developed feelings about the illness, and, quite likely, anxieties about it. Very few people can simply accept that they have an illness without any concern. Of course, that worry puts the person in a frame of mind which then means that they may return to their cognitive interpretation and amend it in line with their concerns. If they are in a lot of pain, which is getting stronger, they might decide to amend the time-line cognition, because they might think that the amount of pain they are experiencing suggests a longer-term illness than they had previously thought. Fear might cause them to choose a more dramatic identity and cause for their illness than is appropriate. Doctors in Accident and Emergency departments are very familiar with people experiencing dyspepsia (indigestion) who think that they might be having a heart attack because both can involve chest pains. Of course, once a person has interpreted the symptoms in this way, things can become complicated. One of the symptoms of anxiety is chest pain, even in those people with a perfectly healthy heart. If the anxiety over believing that the chest pain caused by dyspepsia is actually heart dysfunction causes further chest pain, the situation worsens, and the cognitions that the individual has about what is happening to their body keep on being amended.

The second stage is **coping**. This is where the individual starts to do something about their illness. In a sense, this is the thing we can most easily measure, i.e. health/illness behaviour. Coping can come in two basic forms, dealing with the challenge (**approach coping**), and failing to deal with it or denying it (**avoidance coping**). Examples of approach coping are adopting a different lifestyle, joining self-help groups, carefully complying with advice from a doctor and medication regimens and so on. Avoidance coping involves denying that the illness is present and ignoring the symptoms or amending the cognitions so that the identity of the illness changes to something much more trivial. It also includes, related to this, the concept of **unrealistic optimism**, an idea postulated by Weinstein (1982; 1984). People commonly hold the view that certain diseases will not affect them, even when their genetic and lifestyle characteristics suggest that they will. Similarly, once a disease or illness has begun, an unrealistic optimist is open to cognitions which reflect this. Unreal optimism blended with denial could take the form of avoidance behaviour like saying to oneself (and believing) things like 'I have developed diabetes, but the doctors might be wrong. You hear about tests going wrong all of the time. And even if they are right, I'm sure it'll not affect me. It'll be a really mild form and I will hardly notice it.' Croyle *et al* (1997) categorise these biases in perception into four main camps which, paraphrased, are threat bias ('the disease is not serious'), test bias ('the tests used by the doctors are not reliable'), prevalence bias ('it's a really common disease, so I'm not alone') and time-line bias ('it'll clear up soon').

The third stage of self-regulation is **appraisal** of the coping strategy. This is where a person assesses the coping mechanisms they are using and, depending on the results of their assessment, maintains the behaviour or adopts a new, different coping strategy. There are some problems here for the model, since some research seems to suggest that many people never enter this stage, that is they do not assess their coping strategy, perhaps because they are only open to one type of strategy. This might particularly affect the avoiders, since they perhaps always rely on avoidance, which is more or less the same each time. Also, avoiders will not assess their coping since they do not see their avoidance as a form of coping. They are, after all, in their belief, not ill.

We now turn to a piece of research which has attempted to validate the self-regulatory model. Steed *et al* (1999) focused on atrial fibrillation, a heart condition which predisposes a person to stroke because blood clots are more likely to form. Essentially, Atrial Fibrillation (AF) concerns abnormal heart rhythms. What makes it particularly good to study is that some people have symptoms, such as palpitations and breathlessness, whereas other people do not. Some people have no idea that they have AF until it is diagnosed by their doctor. Most therapeutic measures put into place by doctors aim to reduce the unpleasant symptoms, since AF can seriously affect quality of life. According to the self-regulatory model, representations of illness, and coping, work together to create the overall experience of illness that a person has and their adjustment to their illness. In their sample of 21 females and 41 males, no relationship was found between severity of AF and how people viewed their illness, in all but one of the measures used. This means that people viewed their AF in the same ways, regardless of whether or not they experienced any symptoms. They did not seem to use their symptoms as an indication of the severity of their illness. The authors argue that the main source of information (and thus representations) of their illness comes from doctors, and so this takes over from their own internal monitoring mechanisms.

However, there was a relationship between experiencing symptoms and adjustment to the illness. Contrary to what the self-regulatory model suggests, illness representations and coping did not seem to intervene between experience of symptoms and adjustment. It is as if there is a direct link between symptom experience and adjustment. In fact, there was only a tiny prediction of adjustment based upon coping itself. However, the authors explain these findings mainly by referring to flaws in their design, when actually it is just as likely that the self-regulatory model has shortcomings, especially when applied to certain illnesses and diseases in certain contexts. Like all models, which are essentially theoretical, the realities of illness and the ways that people think about them could be as individualistic as people's tastes in music or their feelings about their friends. By attempting to collect data on groups, we run the risk of missing out on the sometimes contradictory and idiosyncratic nature of any given person's thoughts, feelings and ideas.

WHEN BEHAVIOUR INFLUENCES ATTITUDES

Many models stress the importance of attitudes in shaping behaviour. However, the link between behaviour and attitudes in the other direction has been less well explored. Does doing something lead you to believe that it is a good thing, or at least not a bad thing? Bennett and Clatworthy (1999) demonstrate exactly how this may occur. Theirs was a study of women who smoked during pregnancy. They found that those who continued to smoke whilst carrying a child were less likely to agree with statements that stressed the harm that smoking can do to their baby. However, even these women had reduced the number of cigarettes that they smoked, which seems contradictory given that they deny the harmful effects it may have on their child. The authors suggest that actual dependence on nicotine was an important modifying factor. These women were addicted to nicotine, and so felt that giving up completely was not a viable option for them. Their answer to this was to cut down smoking, rather than cut it out, but to deny the harm it may cause. This can be seen as a protective strategy. Although it does not protect physical health, it may protect mental health because the women concerned do not have to face the stress of knowing that they are smoking but are damaging their baby. By denying the harmful effects, they have let their behaviour shape their attitudes in a way that reduces any contradictions in their life.

CONCLUDING REMARKS

A careful reading of this chapter should reveal that a great many of the theories and models developed in health psychology began life elsewhere, usually in social psychology, and that most models and theories have a remarkable amount in common. At times, the models can seem indistinguishable from each other. Many are developed from each other, hence their similarities. The history of the development of virtually every model or theory in health psychology is one where they have been refined by adding to them, not taking things away. As health psychology evolves, there is every possibility that hybridisation across models will increase, until, rather than seeing a proliferation of models, we will see a gradual reduction in their number, perhaps to one or two models which incorporate many of their forbears and are, perhaps by necessity, rather complicated and multivariate. Simple models are likely to die out, because, as we have noted elsewhere in this book, human behaviour is not simple, and is underpinned by a large number of factors.

Study questions

1. Ask a dozen people, of various ages and backgrounds if possible, what causes the common cold and what can be done to prevent it and to help to cure it. Compare their answers.

2. Is it possible to change someone's beliefs? Can health behaviour be changed without alteration to health beliefs?

FURTHER READING

Conner, M. and Norman, P. (eds) (1995): *Predicting Health Behaviour.* Buckingham: Open University Press. At times heavy going, but a good indicator of the complexities of health cognition and behaviour models applied to particular issues.

Petrie, K.J. and Weinman, J.A. (eds) (1997): *Perceptions of Health and Illness.* Amsterdam: Harwood Academic. Another edited book with chapters on a range of health behaviours and illnesses, showing how health psychologists attempt to understand them.

4 Differences Between People

- Introduction
- Cultural differences
- Gender
- Age
- Intelligence
- Disability
- Locus of control (LoC)
- Challenges to LoC
- Types A and B personality and hostility
- Optimism/pessimism
- Anxiety and neuroticism
- Hypochondriasis
- Adherence and compliance
- Individual differences applied to health professionals
- Concluding remarks
- Study questions
- Further reading

INTRODUCTION

No-one would challenge the assertion that there are different kinds of people in the world. People differ in culture, but also in temperament, sense of humour, confidence, intelligence, and numerous other facets of personality. All of these things can, to some degree, affect health beliefs and health behaviour. A pain in the leg will not mean the same thing to every person, nor will advice from a doctor to 'take a break from work', nor will a diagnosis of a benign pituitary tumour.

Sometimes, taking the average from a group of people spreads out thinly some of the most important trends in the data. The mean average of both of these two sets of numbers (1, 2, 3, 4, 5, 6, 7, 8, 9; 1, 1, 1, 1, 1, 1, 9, 9, 9, 9, 9) is 5. Of course, as you can see, one set is very different from the other. Sometimes those differences are overlooked, wrongly so. The average person is Chinese. It sounds strange, and it is, of course, a pointless thing to say. But statistically it is true, if you use the modal average, because there are more Chinese people on earth than any other grouping. An even more ridiculous statistic would be that the average person is mostly Chinese but quite Indian. Calculating a mean average would lead you to this conclusion, because India has the next largest population after China. Again, it is meaningless.

This chapter takes a look at some of the factors *pertaining to the individual or to groups of individuals with a certain characteristic* that psychologists have researched which can influence health-related behaviours. It is not possible to cover all of the individual differences here, but some of the better-researched topics are detailed.

CULTURAL DIFFERENCES

Both psychologists and sociologists have devoted much attention to the issue of cultural differences, not only in the interpretation of health and illness but in health behaviours and in compliance with medical advice. Only a few studies are mentioned here as examples of that work.

Some of the classic work on cultural differences in health behaviour comes from a sociologist, Zola. Zola (1966) commented on the differences between Irish and Italian Americans in symptom reporting. Italian Americans tended to report a larger number of symptoms. However, Irish Americans were much more likely to present with ear, nose and throat complaints than were Italian Americans. Lipton and Marbach (1984), in their study of facial pain amongst a number of ethnic groupings in America, have found that pain perception is culturally determined.

Sissons Joshi (1995) conducted a study of causal beliefs about insulin-dependent diabetes in both England and India. By asking people what they believed had caused their diabetes, she found some similarities and some differences between the English people and the Indian people. More Indian people blamed their diet than did English people, and far more Indian diabetics believed that eating too much sweet food had been the cause (38% as opposed to 6% of the English sample). Of those patients who said that they had diabetes in the family, only a third of them mentioned heredity as a cause of their disease, in both samples. Most interesting was that some people in both samples were reluctant to think about causality, and this proportion was higher in the Indian sample. The people who could not give a cause for their diabetes in the English sample tended to be those who reported not having adjusted very well to the disease, whereas in the Indian sample adjustment was not related to causal reasoning. This shows that when we construct our models of what people do, and why and how, we must not fall into the trap of believing that a model constructed based on one, culturally biased sample, necessarily holds for the thousands of different groups of people in the world, many of whom live dramatically different lives from the largely middle-class, white, Western researchers.

Zimba and Buggie (1993) demonstrated the power of culture in determining people's health beliefs using an experimental design to ascertain the strength of belief in both orthodox, Western medicine, and traditional African medicines. Twenty-one undergraduates from Malawi were told that they were going to be given a substance intended to arouse the body, thus affecting temperature and pulse. On one day they were given the substance in the form of a traditional. herbal remedy, and on another they were given it in the form of a typical Western medicine. Both affected temperature (but not pulse), and equally. The important factor here is that the substance was merely a placebo. It contained nothing which could have this effect pharmacologically. However, because the students believed that it would affect their body, it did. Importantly, the fact that both worked equally shows that in countries where different types of medicine exist side by side, faith in both can be similar. A similar study conducted in a country where *only* herbal remedies or *only* Western medicines have credibility is unlikely to produce the same results.

A fascinating study of folk illness by Scheper-Hughes (1999) shows that complicated belief systems can arise which are often metaphors for larger social problems. She studied the conception of a folk illness called 'nervoso' in people living in poverty in North-East Brazil. Often, people seemed very preoccupied with the disease, symptoms of which include anger, depression, tremor, weakness, dizziness, and wasting. It is conceptualised as a nervous disease, like having 'bad nerves' in Britain. The 'cures' for nervoso tend to involve various tonics and vitamin drinks, but increasingly drugs such as tranquillisers and sleeping pills. What Scheper-Hughes points out is that people will readily speak of nervoso but not of hunger. For whatever reason, nervoso appears to be a publicly acceptable way to cope with the much greater social problem of starvation, since the symptoms of hunger closely match those of nervoso. People believe in nervoso, despite it being obvious to the outsider that it is really hunger. Scheper-Hughes suggests that it is more than hunger, however, but a metaphor for the social conditions in which these people live. This is, perhaps, why nervoso is so common; everyone lives in the same conditions. What we can learn from this is that entire social groups consisting of a great many people can develop strong belief systems about illness which can be misleading to the outsider and which may be clues to a social problem. In a sense, this is not surprising. The fact that heart disease is common in Britain must tell us something about the practices and eating habits of British people and the ways that they live.

Socio-economic status is a major determinant of health, and tends to be bound up with cultural identity. As such, it is appropriate to consider 'social class' under culture. However, there is always confounding in these studies, since socio-economic status is not something that a person has in isolation from other things. Education, money, social support, self-esteem, and so on influence and are influenced by each other. A middle-class person is likely to have a different pattern of these from a working-class person. All of these things may influence health, indirectly through nutrition, and directly through things such as interaction with the doctor (who, almost by definition, is middle-class).

A special issue of the *Journal of Health Psychology* in 1997 was devoted to socio-economic factors in health. Carroll and Davey Smith (1997) suggest that health psychologists need to be interested in these factors rather than just taking them into account in other studies. They show that health inequalities have always existed, and that they persist even in wealthy groups. The wealthiest of the wealthy have healthier lives than the poorest of the wealthy. It is not just a matter of comparing rich with poor, but richer with poorer. They give some fascinating data on inequalities based upon fatalities when the *Titanic* sunk in 1912. Of women in first-class cabins 2.8% died, compared with 45.3% of women in third-class cabins. The treatment of people is based upon their wealth, and how they are treated can determine their health, or in this case life or death. Cavelaars *et al* (1997) looked at trends in culture and socio-economic status across the European Community, and found that there were substantial differences in smoking behaviour, alcohol consumption, tendency to be overweight and consumption of fresh vegetables from country to country. In general, poorer people (and people from countries with a weaker economy) tended to smoke more, be overweight, eat fewer vegetables and drink more alcohol. The authors suggest that smoking and drinking can be common coping mechanisms for poorer people. They also put forward the idea that availability of fresh vegetables can be restricted in some areas, typically those where poorer people live. However, they note that this is reversed the further south one travels. Therefore, in countries in the South of Europe, poorer people often eat more vegetables than their richer counterparts. One more striking suggestion is that the trend towards obesity in people from lower socio-economic strata can be explained by reference to social mobility. Previous research has shown that people who are overweight are less likely to get better and better jobs and work their way up the social ladder than are leaner people. What Cavelaars *et al* demonstrate is that patterns in health inequalities are seen across cultures, but also within cultures. What explains something in one country does not necessarily explain it in another. For health psychology, an approach which avoids ethnocentrism must be adopted.

GENDER

Men and women are different. If nothing else, there are biological differences. As has been seen in the first chapter, the differences in the biological makeup of men and women can manifest themselves in quite varied behaviours.

Probably as a consequence of intrinsic factors such as the nature of the hormones circulating in the body, and extrinsic factors like socialisation and differential treatment of boys and girls and then men and women in society, men and women have their own specific health problems. Where the sexes share a problem, there are differences in the way that they interpret and cope with that health threat. From a history where there was a disproportionate amount of attention paid to 'male' illness and disease, we have progressed to the point where greater numbers of researchers are looking at male *and* female health.

Pain threshold does not seem to be the same for men and women, nor does pain tolerance. (If you wanted to study pain, from crushing a finger in a vice for instance, threshold would be determined by the pressure at which the person first reports pain and tolerance by how long the person could withstand a given degree of pain. Thus threshold and tolerance interact. Generally, tolerance goes down as threshold goes down; the stronger the stimulus applied, the greater the likelihood that pain is reported, and the shorter time the pain can be withstood.) Experimental studies, where people are artificially subjected to pain in controlled conditions, often show that women have both lower thresholds and lower tolerances for pain compared with men, but some studies show no difference. Others show that women and men differ only in tolerance, rather than both measures (Goolkasian, 1985). Of course, such studies are always confounded by socialisation. In many societies, including those where the research has usually been conducted, there are sex-role differences in expression of emotion. Showing weakness by reporting pain is at odds with the traditional Western concept of masculinity, whereas it partly coincides with the feminine role. Thus, it might not be that women and men feel different amounts of pain when subjected to exactly the same stimulus, but that women are more at liberty to express the pain that they do feel, men being constrained to appear 'tough' and 'strong'. Possible evidence for this comes from Levine and De Simone (1991), who found that the sex of the experimenter interacted with that of the participant. When a woman tests the pain sensitivity of a man, he reports less pain than he would otherwise, but the woman tested by a man reports more pain. The same problems are likely to arise when looking at real-world pain, imposed by disease or illness, and so the results of such work must also be considered with this in mind.

In a study of the common cold, MacIntyre (1993) found that men exaggerated their symptoms more than women. This suggests that women might tolerate physical discomfort more than men, depending on how discomfort is operationally defined. This does not contradict the work that shows that pain threshold and tolerance is lower in women, since common colds, like many illnesses, do not involve significant pain, but instead a constellation of unpleasant bodily symptoms. Women might be more capable than men of coping with illness in its holistic form.

To take another topic in health psychology, one would predict differences between men and women, on average, in dietary behaviour, since the social norms for body image in men and women are quite different. Men seek muscular bodies more than do women, and women seek to be 'slim' more often (Lewis and Blair, 1993). This, however, may be cut across by other factors such as sexuality. Gay men are more likely to experience eating disorders than are straight men, for instance.

AGE

As we age, we change, not only physically but in our abilities to perform tasks and in our attitudes, beliefs and opinions. One rather obvious but overlooked way in which advancing age affects health is in terms of sensory capabilities. Older people tend to have poorer vision, and also a poorer sense of smell (and thus taste). Since these deteriorate very slowly, decrements might not be noticed by people as they age. As a result, older people are less likely to detect if something is wrong with their food. When milk is 'off' we tend to smell that it is. Even if we do not, we certainly taste it if we make the mistake of drinking it. Some older people will not. As a consequence, they may poison themselves. Since immune functioning also declines with age, bacterial poisoning is a much more serious issue for older people than younger ones.

Similarly, some infections generate odours. Intertrigo is a fungal infection of crevices formed when two skin areas meet and moisture builds up. Whilst it is more common in overweight individuals, anyone can develop it, since even the lightest of people have such areas on their body, such as armpits and the groin. Intertrigo can be identified partly because it can be associated with an odour, usually like blue cheese or mushrooms. If an older person has a diminished sense of smell, it might take them longer to notice that something is awry, and thus longer to report this to a doctor.

Lastly, older people are often poorer people. As a result they may eat less healthily and compromise on hygiene in order to save money. The consequences of these behaviours are clear.

INTELLIGENCE

A growing literature exists on intelligence and health beliefs and behaviour, particularly in respect to people with learning disabilities, who are often of lower intelligence than average. Much more research needs to be done, however. Whilst a great deal of health psychology concerns itself with creating models of behaviour based upon rationality and reason, a great many people with learning disabilities have alternative cognitions which do not match those models. People with learning disabilities think differently about things. They may have different values. Kent and Croucher (1998) suggest a number of ways in which dental behaviour can be affected by a learning disability. Such people may have difficulty with the co-ordinated movements of brushing the teeth, or they may forget to brush them altogether. Epilepsy is something which affects a higher proportion of people with learning disabilities than in the remaining population. Such people must care for their teeth well, since they cannot wear dentures because they are unsafe when a person undergoes a seizure. The more one investigates such phenomena, the more details are uncovered which are important to the life of the person concerned but are easily overlooked by psychologists and doctors trying to make a difference.

DISABILITY

One of the growing areas of research, but one which is under-represented in the literature of individual differences at present, is disability. A lot of the work into disability by psychologists has been focused on coping and rehabilitation, therapy and 'cure'. There is, however, a very strong backlash amongst some groups against this medical-model-oriented version of what disability means. Disability need not be defined negatively, in terms of what people can and cannot do, but in terms of a culture, a difference between people rather than a shortcoming in the disabled person. For instance, many deaf people, especially if they use sign language as a first language, see themselves as a linguistic minority, rather like the Spanish-speaking people in New York or the Somalians in London, and may not see themselves as 'disabled' at all. This is the first lesson a psychologist dealing with disabled people should learn; not all people with an impairment are disabled, and not all perceive themselves as disabled.

Health issues within the culture of disability vary from disability to disability, and from person to person. In fact, disability is a perfect example of a difference that highlights the tremendous variation between individuals. Take any of the other factors listed in this chapter as individual differences, and disabled people, obviously, differ along those dimensions as much as do non-disabled people. Johnston (1996; 1997) has aimed to create models to understand disability in a health context. She calls for a view of disability which includes not only the psychosocial consequences of a disability but the emotions and cognitions which may contribute to or diminish that disability. Not all disabled people feel and act in the same way; individual differences between them can make their disability worse or better. Disabled people differ in the same ways as do non-disabled people, and their personalities interact with their disability. We now turn to some of those characteristics which health psychologists have identified.

LOCUS OF CONTROL (LoC)

Since Rotter (1966) first published details of his theory of locus of control (LoC) and a method of measuring it, a great deal of research has been directed towards elucidating this concept. It is a simple idea, but it has spawned so much research that it can clearly be identified as one of the key constructs in health psychology.

Locus of control is a term used to describe the basic view that a person has about things that happen to them. Some people tend to think that they are responsible for things that happen to them, and some people tend to think that they are not. Some people blame themselves for events which occur in their lives, and some people prefer to blame external factors, such as fate or chance. Some people feel that they can control their lives, others do not. According to Rotter, those people who feel in charge of their lives have an **internal locus of control**, and those who feel more at the mercy of others or of chance have an **external locus of control**. The consequences of this for health behaviours are obvious. If you believe that you can influence what happens in your life, you are likely to believe that you can make a difference to your health if you try. If you are more fatalistic, you are much less likely to try to change things, including your current health status. Not surprisingly, when the notion of LoC is applied to health it is called **health locus of control**.

Over time it became clear that this dualistic version of LoC was, perhaps, too simplistic. As research into LoC progressed, Levenson (1974) pointed out that there was a substantial difference between those externals who felt that mainly chance factors were responsible for life events and those who said that the influence of other people on their lives was most significant. Thus, a splitting of the external locus of control was effected. People who were previously lumped together as externals were now seen as having an external locus directed at either **powerful others** or **chance**.

As LoC was applied to health it was a matter of time before a specific instrument to measure it in a health context was developed. The Multi-dimensional Health Locus of Control Scale (Wallston *et al*, 1978) does just this. This, and other scales like it (such as that of Lau and Ware, 1981), resemble the standard LoC measurement instruments, but with questions which clearly assess health-related control. The items pick up who the person feels is responsible for their health, using words like 'blame' and 'fault' and 'fate', and so the purpose is relatively transparent to the respondent.

Research into the health LoC construct has generated some very mixed results. Even with a fixed area of study, such as predicting smoking cessation or alcohol abuse using LoC, varied results have been obtained. Sometimes LoC does assist in the prediction of various health behaviours, and sometimes it does not. Even contradictory results have been obtained.

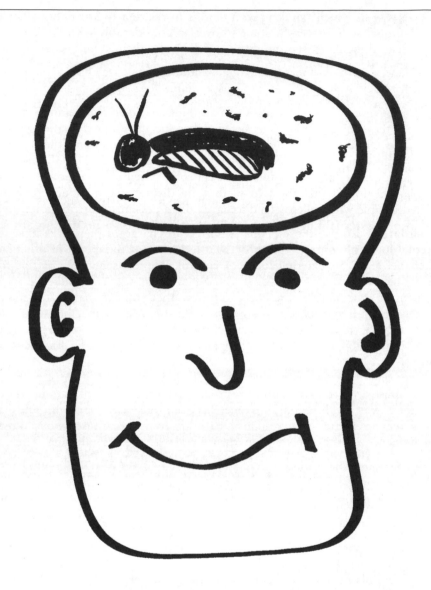

THE PSYCHOLOGIST SAID THAT I SHOULD BE OKAY AS LONG AS I KEEP MY INTERNAL LOCUSTS IN CONTROL

One way in which LoC has been used is in relation to attributional style. Attributional style is seen by some to overlap considerably with LoC, and at times it is difficult to see the difference between them. One useful way to distinguish between them is to see attributional style as a perception of the cause of events, and LoC as the perception of the control a person has over future events and what happens to them. So, a person with a pessimistic attributional style sees the causes of bad things as fixed, stable and general, whereas they see good things as being rather specific and external. A person with an external LoC feels that whatever the cause of something, they are not able to affect the outcome of it by their own actions. Gehlert (1996) looked at both factors in relation to adults with epilepsy, based upon a sample of 144 people. She found that the two factors are distinct, even though they are related. People with epilepsy tend to have both a pessimistic attributional style and also an external LoC. This should be no surprise. It means that, rightly so, they see their epilepsy as stable and as coming from inside of themselves, and which they did not cause. Also, they do not view themselves as being particularly able to do much about their epilepsy in the future, instead feeling that, for instance, powerful others such as doctors can exert influence over it using drugs and so on. It is difficult to argue with this point of view.

CHALLENGES TO LoC

There are, as you would expect, problems with the construct of LoC. The main one is that people are not necessarily always internalisers or externalisers. People switch their locus depending upon the context and the questions asked. They might also change their LoC as they age, depending on life experiences. A person who, when younger, had an internal LoC, but who had a number of experiences which created a sense of powerlessness, where their attempts to influence and direct their life met with failure (either perceived or actual), might slowly drift towards an external LoC, justifying this by believing that their original model of how the world works was naïve. Conversely, it is possible that some people who have an ostensibly external LoC do so as a strategy of coping. In reality, their external locus might be a form of denial. They might blame others rather than face their own responsibilities. Over time, they might learn to take more responsibility in life, for whatever reason, and so become more internalistic.

Another problem concerns what is called **health value**. This, simply, is the value that people put upon their health. Wallston and Wallston (1980) point out that LoC can really only be a predictor of behaviour when people actually value their health. Not everyone thinks that it is important to be healthy. If you are one of those people who do not, you may be unlikely to try to change your behaviours even if you are an internaliser.

These criticisms of health LoC suggest that it is, perhaps, of limited use in predicting health behaviours, especially when employed as a single measure. In recent years, research into health LoC has tailed off somewhat, perhaps reflecting the chequered history it has had.

TYPES A AND B PERSONALITY AND HOSTILITY

Another dimension along which people can vary is described using the terms **Type A** and **Type B** personality. Type A behaviour is associated, it is claimed, with an increased risk of coronary heart disease (CHD), and Type B, associated with a lower risk. First suggested by Friedman and Rosenman (1959; 1974), this dimension of personality is best summarised by descriptions of Type A and Type B 'people' (Types A and B are strictly descriptions of behaviour, but for ease they are often referred to as descriptions of people with that behaviour).

- **Type A:** a typical Type A person is prone to talking loudly and quickly, interrupting others, impatience, competitiveness and hostility. The Type A person does not like to wait for things to happen, they tend to take work very seriously, they do not like queuing, they prefer action to inaction. They do not tolerate others very well.
- **Type B:** a Type B person is simply a person who does not act like a Type A person. Thus they are generally more relaxed, easy-going, softly spoken, co-operative and philanthropic.

Research into this personality factor has produced very mixed results. Whilst some studies have shown evidence that CHD is correlated with Type A behaviour, others have not, particularly those conducted more recently. Because of the mixed results, it became clear that we would need to refine our models and look more closely at the behaviours which make up Type A to see if only *some* of those behaviours are really predictive of CHD. Hostility has been a characteristic carefully focused on. Hostility can be described as a non-specific dislike of others, a tendency towards seeing the worst in other people's behaviour, and lack of compassion. It tends to have three facets, behavioural, emotive and cognitive. The behavioural aspect is demonstrated through aggression and, possibly, bullying, the cognitive through (for example) mistrust of others, and the emotive through anger and envy. In a meta-analysis of the literature on CHD and hostility, Miller *et al* (1996) conclude that there is a good relationship between them. These authors suggest that social support may be a key factor linking hostility and poor health. It is established that social support is a significant influence on health. If we have the support of important people in our lives, friends, family, perhaps even wider society, then we are more likely to be healthy and more likely to be restored to health quickly should anything go awry. Of course, hostile individuals may lack social support precisely because they are hostile. They dislike other people, leading other people to dislike them. Probably a confounding factor is the health-related behaviour of hostile individuals. They have an enhanced tendency to perform injurious acts to health, such as avoiding exercise and drinking alcohol to excess (Houston and Vavak, 1991). Thus we can see that the simple Type A/Type B distinction fails to take into account other factors, both in personality and behaviour, which can lead to the type of disposition which may be a risk factor in CHD.

OPTIMISM/PESSIMISM

The extent to which someone is optimistic, whether rightly or wrongly so, can influence their interpretations and behaviour. It is appropriate to distinguish between realistic and unrealistic optimism.

Realistic optimism would involve a sensible set of cognitions and beliefs about the prognosis of the disease, focusing on the better outcomes associated with the disease. Not all cancers kill people, and if someone has a type of cancer which is fatal only half of the time then focusing on the 50% chance that they will survive rather than the 50% chance that they will die might be seen as a realistic form of optimism. (Pessimism, of course, would involve focusing on the 50% chance of death.) Optimism is good for people who are ill, at least in Scheier and Carver's (1985) view, because optimists strive to achieve their goals since they see them as attainable. Striving (as opposed to not striving) enhances success, since some of the time the attempts to achieve goals will pay off. Pessimists may not choose to make an effort since they may believe that their efforts will be wasted. (Note the remarkable similarity between optimistic thinking and internal LoC.) Optimism which is part of someone's nature is referred to as **dispositional optimism**. Scheier and colleagues (Scheier *et al*, 1994) have devised and revised a short, ten-item test of dispositional optimism called the Life Orientation Test (LOT). Research into the moderating effects of dispositional optimism has demonstrated some interesting results. It seems that optimists recover more quickly from coronary bypass surgery than pessimists (Scheier *et al*, 1989). They also have a better quality of life six months after the surgery. Work-in-progress reported by Leventhal *et al* (1997) suggests that pessimists and optimists differ in their ability to judge their vulnerability to health problems. In a study of over five years, pessimists and optimists were asked to rate their health and then monitored over the years. As you would imagine, the optimists rated their health as better than the pessimists did. More interestingly, the pessimists claiming to have excellent health were compared with those claiming to have poor health, with the same comparison being made in optimists. Death rates amongst the sample were then looked at. 'Poor health optimists' were only 1.5 times more likely to have died than 'excellent health optimists', showing that, perhaps, the optimists who thought that their health was good were actually being too optimistic! However, 'poor health pessimists' were more than seven times likely to have died than 'excellent health pessimists'. This demonstrates that when a pessimist rates their health as poor, they tend to be closer to reality than anyone, or, equally, that when a pessimist believes that they have poor health, this belief, coupled with a pessimistic disposition, is more likely to lead to negative health outcomes and even death.

Unrealistic optimism is the state where a person believes that they are not susceptible to a disease when they actually are, despite evidence to the contrary, and where, if they have contracted an illness, they believe that theirs will be shorter and less severe than it is likely to be in reality. It is based on the work of Weinstein (1982; 1984). Because unrealistic optimists believe that they will be fine, they may underestimate their need for coping. This, in a sense, is where the danger comes in, since they will fail to develop appropriate behaviour in dealing with their illness or in preventing an illness occurring. Unlike the dispositional optimist, they do not set goals which correspond to the reality of the situation, and so are not taking practical steps to either avoid illness or eradicate it. In fact, unrealistic optimists are open to the added danger of creating or exacerbating illness by engaging in damaging behaviours which they believe are safe because they do not feel at risk from health problems.

ANXIETY AND NEUROTICISM

The extent to which people are 'natural worriers' can have a significant impact on their mental and physical health. The anxiety feeds into health, and health into anxiety, in a fully reciprocal way. If a woman misses a period, the more she worries about it the greater the risk that she will delay the period further. A man who worries about pain focuses on the pain, and as a result the pain feels stronger. Stronger pain worries him even more, and so on.

Although psychologists do distinguish between anxiety and neuroticism, both are examples of behaviour which produces similar outcomes. Also, neurotic people do tend to worry more (be more anxious). The two are related. Psychologists like to keep them separate because anxiety is a state whereas neuroticism is a personality trait. Thus, anxiety can affect all of us in the appropriate circumstances, and is unlikely to last long, whereas neuroticism is a characteristic of only some of us, but tends to last a lifetime. Typically, neurotic people tend to report more symptoms than those who are less neurotic, but do not necessarily have more health problems. Thus neurotic people, because they tend to be very circumspect and mentally active, notice what is happening to their bodies in fine detail and so have a heightened sensitivity to bodily change (Watson and Pennebaker, 1989). Twinges of pain, creaking joints, occasional dizziness, mood swings, digestive problems, mouth ulcers, headaches and the like are quite normal experiences and are generally part of the successful functioning of the bodily systems. Even the healthiest of people experience them from time to time. The body is like a house. Sometimes you hear noises in the night, but it does not mean that there is any need to be alarmed. Neurotic people will tend to be alarmed, however, and just as they might be unable to sleep after hearing a creaking floorboard or branches tapping on a window in the wind, so they will also worry unduly because they experience normal phenomena within the body which other people would not be perturbed by or perhaps not even notice.

HYPOCHONDRIASIS

Hypochondriasis (*not* hypochondria, as it is often mistakenly abbreviated to) is the name given to the state of being unduly anxious about one's health, often to the point where the obsession starts to have a disabling effect on the individual's life. Extreme hypochondriacs are few and far between (the kind of people who need help because they truly believe that they are constantly ill and are frightened to involve themselves in the outside world for fear of illness and disease), but a mild degree of hypochondriasis is present in many people. Most of us know or have known someone with a preoccupation with aches and pains and, perhaps, excessive interest in hygiene. It is commonly reported that many medical students display signs of hypochondriasis by feeling like they have developed or are developing many of the health problems which they are studying, sometimes called **medical students' disease** (Woods *et al*, 1966).

Hypochondriasis is of great interest to psychologists because it is entirely psychological. By definition, it is about people who *think* that they are ill, and not about people who actually are. It is essentially the opposite of denial, one might argue (Antonovsky and Hartman, 1974), since in denial people who are ill believe that they are not, whereas in hypochondriasis people who are not ill believe that they are. People who are neurotic or anxious tend to be more hypochondriacal. In health belief terms, the hypochondriac tends to have an overly high fear of a disease in addition to believing that they have it (Kellner, 1985). Hypochondriacs do not, usually, present to a doctor with concerns over a disease which does not frighten them. They might have some genuine physical disease, however, but their concern over it will far outstrip the seriousness of it and they may have misrepresented the symptoms of a mild problem as signs of some fatal disease.

Hypochondriacs often believe they have developed symptoms of currently 'famous' diseases (Warwick and Salkovskis, 1990). When AIDS first began to come to public awareness, and the media ran scare stories, this was a popular focus for hypochondriacs. Two extreme British cases of this are reported by Miller *et al* (1985). These patients, who strongly believed despite doctors' protestations to the contrary that they had AIDS, were significantly affected mentally. This is in line with the legendary stories of medical students expressing anxiety over problems they have recently studied. The short-term solution to hypochondriacal fears is advice and reassurance, from doctors ideally, but from significant others in addition. Short-term is the key here, since as Salkovskis and Warwick (1986) point out, the person becomes 'addicted', in a sense, to the reassurance, which then is likely to become problematic *per se* and certainly does not assist in reducing either the level of anxiety over health or the hypochondriasis in general. There is another problem here which should be expressed. When a doctor tells a patient that there is 'nothing wrong' with them, this will not be reassuring and comforting in all cases. If a person truly believes that something is wrong, and has experienced symptoms which are real to them, then being told that nothing is wrong seems like a mistaken conclusion. They are more likely to believe that the doctor is wrong, and, therefore, take up more resources seeking further medical opinions.

Ferguson (1996) tried to relate knowledge about medical matters to hypochondriasis, comparing medical students' disease to lay hypochondriasis. Knowledge of four types was assessed in 58 undergraduate participants: anatomy, vital signs (blood pressure and pulse), disease aetiology and disease symptomatology. A distinction was made between actual knowledge and perceived knowledge (what people know and what they *think* that they know expressed as a function of confidence in their knowledge). The accuracy with which people can judge their knowledge is known as **calibration**. Ferguson found that the more people knew about the causes of disease the more they felt at risk from them and sought reassurance that they were healthy. However, those people most concerned about their bodies were those who knew least about anatomy. Therefore, some forms of medical knowledge seem to actually guard against hypochondriacal fears. Looking at calibration, on the other hand, there was a relationship between bodily knowledge and bodily concerns, with those people who were unrealistically confident about what they knew being the most anxious about their bodies. Therefore, the amount of knowledge a person possesses about medical matters is related to their degree of susceptibility to hypochondriasis (or at least, medical students' disease), but the extent to which they are accurate in judging what they know mediates in this relationship. Of course, clinically diagnosed hypochondriacs may or may not show a similar pattern of behaviours to the volunteer undergraduates in Ferguson's study.

Stereotypically, hypochondriacs are seen as neurotic people who pester doctors and waste their time. However, if people behave this way, then they are surely experiencing a health problem in its own right and therefore require some kind of assistance, psychological or otherwise. To reserve health care for those people who really do have an illness is to show a lack of understanding of the extent to which psychological factors influence health. Whether hypochondriacs are encouraged by 'better safe than sorry' health campaigns and policies which tell people to see their doctor if they are worried about their health, remains to be seen.

One further point: the term 'heartsink patient' is used often by doctors to describe the patient who presents regularly and for whom there is often nothing the doctor can do, usually because there is nothing physically wrong with them. The term is taken from the fact that the doctor's heart sinks when the patient turns up, i.e. they feel depressed, helpless, and defeated (Butler and Evans, 1999). This shows clearly how doctors' reactions to patients are important, and that it is not just that doctors can put patients into unpleasant moods but that it is a two-way process.

ADHERENCE AND COMPLIANCE

When doctors and other health professionals give advice, or recommend a specific treatment such as a drug, some people do what they have suggested, and some do not. The terms **adherence** and **compliance** refer to the act of following the advice given. Many authors now prefer the term adherence over compliance, because compliance implies 'giving in' to something, whereas adherence implies 'sticking to' something. Since the treatment of illness is increasingly seen as a collaboration between doctor and patient, rather than the application of a treatment, by a doctor, to a passive and willing patient, adherence is a more suitable term.

There are factors in adherence behaviour which apply not only to patients but also to doctors. The behaviour of a doctor can determine adherence as much as the intentions, values, or personality of the patient. The interaction between health professional and patient is often what determines adherence. However, once a diagnosis has been made and a treatment prescribed a patient is often left on their own to determine the course of their illness. Adherence then depends upon the interpretation that a person makes about their illness, their treatment, and their symptoms. Siegel *et al* (1999) examined drug-schedule adherence in middle-aged and older HIV-infected people. In order to prevent the development of AIDS itself, a combination of anti-viral drugs is prescribed. These researchers aimed to work out what made some people stick to this regime, and what made others depart from it. From interviews they discovered that symptoms often acted as a trigger for non-adherence. Once taking the drugs, people would question their efficacy and safety if they noticed unusual symptoms. If these symptoms were perceived as negative side effects of the medication, then the conditions were ripe for non-adherence. Failure of a drug or combination to ameliorate symptoms was also interpreted negatively.

So, if a treatment seems to be doing nothing, or doing something negative, people stop adhering to it. This is particularly problematic for doctors, since two issues need to be considered. Firstly, people cannot always trust their perceptions. Because a drug *seems* to be doing nothing doesn't mean that it is. Just because a person develops an unpleasant symptom after taking a drug doesn't mean that the drug is responsible for it. We know enough about misperceptions and misattributions in psychology to appreciate this. Secondly, drugs can sometimes take a while to start working. People often expect immediate or quick effects, and many drugs cannot work this way. People also mistakenly believe that when a problem *appears* to have cleared up, then it has. It is common for people taking antibiotics to stop when the symptoms have gone away, or for people using anti-fungal creams for foot infections like *tinea pedis* to do the same. Of course, what happens is that the remaining bacteria or fungi responsible for the problem are given a respite, and they recover their strength and start to attack the body again. Much of what happens to the body is not visible. Symptoms are often the last stage in a long process. Careful education of patients as to exactly what to expect from a treatment can improve adherence, especially in cases where non-adherence stems from lack of knowledge rather than rebelliousness *per se*.

It is not possible in a book of this size to go into detail about the issue of adherence. Books have been written on this topic alone. It is a key issue, and you are recommended to read more about this if you wish to take your study of health psychology further.

INDIVIDUAL DIFFERENCES APPLIED TO HEALTH PROFESSIONALS

Until now, we have concentrated on factors which can vary between patients, and the effects these may have on health behaviours, health values, and treatment received or adhered to. However, it is easy to forget that health professionals are also people who vary along these dimensions. We cannot assume that age, gender, culture, socio-economic background, politics, LoC, neuroticism and many other things do not make a difference to a doctor and their behaviour towards patients. We all know that doctors vary in their personalities; this is self-evident. Of course, accepting this means that we must accept that those personalities will interact with those of the patients in creating the healthcare dynamic. However, almost all research in health psychology until quite recently has focused on the patient's characteristics, rather than those of the healthcare provider. One must remember that doctors may not always be open to being researched, especially when the research aims to identify how their characteristics could be detrimental to a patient's health.

It has long been suggested that doctors in various specialities differ in their personalities. This means, of course, that the type of person you deal with depends upon what your medical condition actually is. McManus *et al* (1996) investigated personality and speciality preference in a large sample of applicants to medical school. By studying applicants rather than the doctors themselves, they were able to rule out the possibility that personalities develop along particular lines as a result of specific training. They found that an interest in entering psychiatry was associated with a measure of fantasy (relating to fictional characters), perspective-taking (being able to think like another person to understand them) and with a measure of unease in difficult social situations. There was no relationship between interest in psychiatry and the extent to which a person feels empathy for others. This was an important variable with respect to general practice and geriatric medicine. Surgeons are people, it seems, who like making things, and are quite sporty. Whilst this might seem a quite frivolous study, it shows that certain types of people are drawn to certain specialities within medicine. It suggests that clusters of personality types will be found in particular departments, in keeping with the saying 'birds of a feather flock together'. Whether this is a good or a bad thing for patients remains to be seen.

CONCLUDING REMARKS

There are a wide range of characteristics of the individual which can contribute to health behaviour and to illness. A health psychologist should try to bear all of these factors in mind when investigating any issue of health. To neglect individual differences can lead to a very distorted picture of what is going on. No single factor should be considered without reference to the others, no matter how cumbersome that might be. The factors can interact, and do. A proper understanding of perceptions, beliefs and behaviours should take a number of variables into account.

No two people are alike. If we want to know why people are different, we need to examine the behaviours (for example) of a middle-class, American, straight, black, Type A, disabled, male with an internal LoC and a middle-class, white, non-disabled, Icelandic gay male with an external LoC, moderate Type A behaviour and some hypochondriasis. Constructing models for behaviour of people at this microscopic level is a challenge for health psychology, but one which it perhaps must face as the discipline develops.

Study questions

1. List as many ways as possible in which people can differ. Try to find at least one way in which each can influence health and health behaviour.

2. Can hypochondriasis create health problems? Who for?

FURTHER READING

Lippa, R.A., Martin, L.R. and Friedman, H.S. (2000): Gender-related individual differences and mortality in the Terman longitudinal study: Is masculinity hazardous to your health? *Personality and Social Psychology Bulletin*, **26**, 1560–70.
   An interesting paper, suggesting that dying younger is associated with higher levels of masculine traits, in both men and women.
Lupton, D. (1994): *Medicine as Culture: Illness, Disease and the Body in Western Societies*. London: Sage.
   A largely sociological account of individual differences and culture in health. Useful for taking a sideways glance at what health psychology does and could involve.

5 Stress and Health

INTRODUCTION

Stress is, arguably, the most researched and documented area of health psychology. To many health psychologists, stress and its sequelae are the main areas of interest for them, professionally. Stress is caused by so many things, and affects just about everything one can imagine. Take any medical condition, and stress will probably have been shown to exacerbate it. Efforts to combat stress represent a massive industry around the world, of which health psychology is a tiny part. Probably the biggest sector of this industry is the sale of 'stress-busting' books, relaxation tapes, exercise routines, and the like. Stress affects probably every person on earth at some point, and is a permanent underlying factor in the lives of many people. You will probably know some people who have experienced heart disease, some cancer, and so on. However, have you ever known anyone who would say that they have never experienced stress? Stress also is unusual in that it can cause itself. If you are aware of your stress symptoms, they are quite likely to increase your stress. Thus, a cycle which is difficult to break can be established.

Mechanic (1978) pointed out that stress can lead to increased use of healthcare resources, not only because stress genuinely causes ill-health, but also because stressed people are more worried and concerned about their health, even when they need not be. A slight pain can seem more serious to a stressed person. Mood is known to have a significant effect on the reporting of symptoms. Someone who is in a negative mood is more likely to report pain, for instance, than a happier person. Salovey and Birnbaum (1989) studied people with influenza or influenza symptoms and used a short procedure to alter their mood experimentally. The people put into a negative mood reported twice as many aches and pains as those in the positive or neutral mood conditions. More pain, or at least more perceived pain, means a greater strain on resources.

We have seen elsewhere, in the chapter on biology and physiology, what the physical effects of stress are, and explored the reasons why the stress response might exist in organisms. Stress leads to increased heart rate, and hypertension. Hypertension is implicated strongly in, for example, deaths from cardio-vascular disease. Thus, stress is a serious issue for study. Here we concentrate on the psychological research into its direct effects on the lives of people, and how stress can be ameliorated.

MEASURING STRESS

A great deal of effort has been put into measuring and cataloguing stress. There are many stress scales in existence, and one of the earliest and most famous attempts to do both came from Holmes and Rahe (1967). They gave a large number of participants a list of things which occur in everyday life, and asked them to rate them as to how difficult it would be for a person to adjust to them. The implication, of course, was that the more stressful something was the more difficult it would be to adjust to. The list of potential stressors included death of a partner, moving house, going to jail, experiencing Christmas, and becoming pregnant. By averaging over the responses, a points system was developed, such that each stressor in a person's life was attached to a certain number of points. By adding up the points, one could see how much stress a person was undergoing. This rather crude approach was soon criticised. Firstly, no attempt was made to build in a factor to account for the differences between individuals. Death of a partner was listed as the most stressful of events, gaining a score of 100 points. However, your age and your partner's age, and the nature of your relationship, and the reason for death, can all interact to affect the level of stress perceived by the individual. In addition, the additive nature of the scale meant that experiencing a set of difficulties often added up to a stress level equivalent to experiencing one major stressor. For example, moving to a smaller house (25 points) and changing one's eating habits (15 points) is as stressful, therefore, as becoming pregnant (40 points). Naturally, such statistical phenomena have little credence for the real people to whom these things are happening. Finally, a significant drawback of the **Social Readjustment Rating Scale (SRRS)** is that it fails to make allowance for the world of difference between a positive and a negative stressor. Going on holiday is stressful, true, but it is also something people want. The same thing applies to moving house. Then there are those stressors which can be positive or negative depending upon the circumstances: some people are glad to be pregnant, others are not; some people are devastated by divorce, others celebrate. However, the SRRS set the agenda for health psychologists to develop more sophisticated tools for the description and measurement of stress.

Life is made up of 'big things' that happen to us, and 'little things'. Ask yourself how many big things happen to you in a year, and then think about how many little things happen. No matter how you choose to define 'big' and 'little', you will probably have to admit that very few big things happen, but that it is perhaps impossible to count all of the little things. A great deal of our stress comes from the little things that happen. Think about how often you find yourself thinking or saying something like 'that bugs me', 'it really winds me up', 'how annoying!' or 'that gets on my nerves'. Kanner *et al* (1981) developed the **Hassles Scale** to try to measure stress caused by little things. Stress from these minor stressors could add up to a significant health problem. They might include having to queue at the bank, feeling fat, waiting for a friend to call, wishing that you could give up smoking, arguing with a family member, or any number of other possibilities. Of course, life isn't just made up of negative things; good things happen too. Because life is a mixture of good things and bad things, sometimes the bad things do not feel quite so bad because a good thing happened. Kanner *et al*, therefore, included a second scale in their study, measuring what they called 'uplifts'. By taking into account scores from both, it was hoped that a better overall picture of experienced stress can be painted. People were given these instruments along with measures of psychological factors such as depression and anxiety. The authors found that hassles were much better predictors of psychological health than were major events, over a period of nine months.

One of the problems with the measurement of daily hassles as an index of stress is of a 'chicken or egg' nature. Daily hassles might be stress in themselves, but equally they might be perceived as stressful only because the person is already stressed by something else (which would have to be some major life event, as measured by Holmes and Rahe). Therefore, major life events may be the main determinant of stress, and daily hassles might simply follow from that. That is, daily hassles are not particularly stressful in themselves, but they may have much greater impact when the person is already stressed. Kanner *et al* (1981) performed a statistical technique to determine this, and discovered that even after major life events had been taken out of the equation, minor events like hassles still predicted psychological health. Therefore, a combination of major and minor stressors, 'softened' if you like by pleasurable and relaxing experiences, seem to determine our stress status.

COPING WITH STRESS

Coping with stress is no different from coping with anything else, in that the ability to do so depends upon both physical and mental resources, and the culture and personality of the individual. Coping is an interesting phenomenon, since it can be a form of cure. In physical injury, such as a broken leg, successful coping will possibly have a small impact on the healing of the bone (via the immune system), but nothing more. However, coping with stressors is quite different. By coping with a stressor, a person removes its label as a stressor. Of course, if something isn't a stressor, it can't cause stress. A lot depends upon how we appraise a situation. Lazarus (1966) developed a transactional model of stress which featured appraisal itself as a process which occurs in two stages (see Fig. 5.1). Primary appraisal is the perception of an event as being either mainly harmful or harmless. Secondary appraisal is the individual's perception of their self-efficacy in dealing with the potential stressor. Events are therefore 'filtered'. Only if an event is perceived as being potentially harmful, and if the person also believes that they are ill-equipped to deal with it, will it become a threat to the individual and be likely to cause full-blown stress. Thus, by dealing with a stressful situation, or coping, it is possible to 'cure' the problem. In the case of non-physical difficulties, coping *is* the cure.

In an important paper for the history of health psychology, Folkman *et al* (1986) set out eight types of coping strategy employed by individuals facing stress.

- **Escape–avoidance:** just as it sounds, this involves 'escapism'. The person tries to avoid the problem by thinking about other things, or by drinking alcohol 'to forget', or by having unrealistic fantasies about magical or lucky ways out of the situation. The person who is about to lose their house because they have been unable to pay the mortgage on account of having been made redundant may decide that they feel happier when drunk, or they may spend time daydreaming about being offered a great job or about winning a lottery. Another common avoidance strategy is to 'throw oneself into one's work'.
- **Distancing:** here, coping involves putting the problem at a metaphorical distance, which can be achieved in a number of ways. Humour is one approach: making the problem into a joke. Another is essentially denial, that is trying not to think about something, as if it hadn't happened.
- **Positive reappraisal:** this is about finding some good in the bad. Experiences are reframed so that the positive in them is identified and focused on. Therefore, people say things like 'losing my sight has done me good because I have put my life into perspective' or 'without losing my baby I would not have realised that other people needed my help and started to work for a charity'.

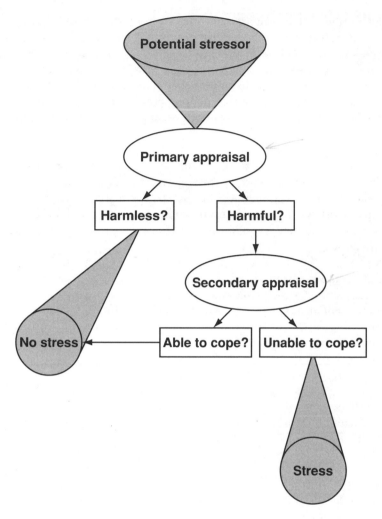

Fig. 5.1 According to Lazarus (1966) two stages of appraisal determine stress

- **Self-controlling:** as you would expect, this involves keeping feelings controlled internally, without seeking external help. It can involve 'bottling up' feelings rather than sharing them, and not showing others that stress is being experienced.
- **Seeking social support:** coping, for some people, is about sharing problems. In contrast with the person who 'bottles up', others prefer to 'get things off their chest'. Thus, seeking social support is a central coping strategy for

many people. They want to tell others about their problems, because it makes them feel better. The English proverb 'A problem shared is a problem halved' demonstrates the pervasiveness of this approach.

- **Planful problem-solving:** a rather obvious strategy, this is about planning a way out of a problem. Whilst it may seem to many to be the first step when a person is in trouble, a lot of people simply do not use this approach, preferring instead to avoid problems or expect fate or their God to help them.

- **Accepting responsibility:** in many ways, it is a healthy approach to accept responsibility for one's actions, and therefore one's problems. Many problems are brought on by a person's own thoughts and actions. However, not all are, and sometimes we are simply unlucky or the victims of the actions of others. Accepting responsibility is not a good strategy when a person is not actually responsible. In these circumstances it is likely to engender negative feelings and to affect self-esteem.

- **Confronting:** this involves dealing with the problem, or the source or creator of the problem, 'head on'. If the bank is threatening to foreclose a loan, speaking to the bank manager, rather than drinking to forget or keeping feelings secret, is a sensible form of confronting. Do not mistake 'confronting' for 'confrontation' or aggression; not all confronting is aggressive, although much of it can be.

Most coping behaviour falls into one or more of these categories. They are not exclusive. Because a person uses one strategy does not mean that they will not use others, even when strategies may give rise to contradictory cognitions. There is nothing to stop a person thinking contradictory things, and most of us do at some time in our lives. Therefore, a stressor may lead to a combination of coping strategies being employed, sometimes confronting, sometimes escape–avoidant. Because someone wants to face a problem today does not mean that they will choose to do the same tomorrow: tomorrow they may prefer to hide away from it by going on holiday or working a long day. Another important consideration is the fact that different stressors may require different approaches, and a person who is typically fixed in a restricted range of strategies may have difficulties coping with stressors of varying nature. The planful, accepting-responsibility or confrontative strategies are particularly useful when a person can actually *do* something about the problem. If they are stressed by noisy neighbours, for instance, there are social and, ultimately, legal ways to deal with this. However, such strategies might be less useful when a person is powerless to change or affect the stressor. If someone loses a leg due to bone cancer they are unlikely to be able to accept responsibility for it themselves, may have no-one to confront, and certainly cannot make plans which will change the fact that they have lost a leg. Admittedly, they can plan for the future and work on living a full life from this moment on, but the fact that the leg has been lost remains. In such a case, seeking social support, positive appraisal and distancing via humour might be more salient techniques of coping.

Sometimes one action or behaviour can be seen as an example of more than one type of coping strategy, calling this division into eight categories into question. You may have heard of individuals who, upon receiving a diagnosis, become fascinated by their illness and read up on it. They become an expert on their illness, and perhaps are able to give advice to others. They may work for or establish some self-help group or charity, and some take to researching the issue, perhaps achieving qualifications on the matter. This, indeed, is known as **intellectualisation** of the illness. Looking at Folkman *et al*'s (1986) division into types of strategy, intellectualisation seems to span more than one of them. It is clearly a distancing approach, looking at the illness as a thing 'out there' to be studied, rather than a property of the person themselves. It is also, perhaps, positive reappraisal, since becoming an expert on an illness is not perceived as a negative thing at all. It might also be confrontive coping, because the person is dealing with the issue head on and, perhaps, confronting others to fight for rights, research monies and so on. Ultimately, this approach could also be seen as long-term planning. If a person seeks to help others (and themselves) through research and knowledge, this is a planful strategy. In addition, social support is sought and perhaps set up via this mode of action, especially if the individual establishes or attends self-help groups and, perhaps, taps into these for purposes of research. The person who tackles the illness in this way also accepts responsibility: they might be seen as saying 'if anyone ought to try to help people with this illness, I as a sufferer ought to' and 'if you want something doing, do it yourself'.

In addition to the above taxonomy, the categories can be further labelled as either **emotion-focused** or **problem-focused**. They are what they sound like: problem-focused coping involves dealing with the problem itself, whereas emotion-focused coping is centred on the emotional reaction to the problem. Self-control, positive appraisal and accepting responsibility, escape–avoidance and distancing are seen as emotion-focused, whereas planful problem-solving and confrontive coping are forms of problem-focused approach. Seeking social support is unusual in that it can be both emotional-focused (in that it is about sharing feelings) and problem-focused (in that it is a way of getting advice about dealing with the problem).

What we must not lose sight of is that coping is also something that doctors have to do. They must deal with death, suffering, clinical error, ethical judgement, failures to save life and so on, every day. They work long hours. Stress is a fact of life for many health professionals, and the coping mechanisms which apply to their patients also apply to them. Medical students and doctors have been known to make jokes about disease and death which some people would regard as highly distasteful. By doing this, they are using distance coping.

Nolen-Hoeksema *et al* (1997) identify two other classifications of coping, this time clearly based in the personalities of the individuals themselves. Copers can be **ruminators,** or **non-ruminators.** In their study of people who had experienced the death of their partner, they found that some people tended to 'chew over' (hence 'ruminate') their grief without achieving anything. They would comment on their thoughts and feelings, repeating stressful assertions without really dealing with them in any way, almost as if describing someone else's thoughts rather than their own. Ruminators, typically, will repeat phrases such as 'I'm not a lucky person. I feel terrible. I can't seem to get right. I don't get better. It seems unfair. I can't really shed this gloom. Why is that?' without really trying to find answers for the questions they generate. In contrast, non-ruminators create plans for dealing with their problems, and work through difficulties with a view to changing things. Ruminators are more likely to experience longer periods of depression or grief following the loss of a partner. Whether ruminators can be successfully taught or encouraged to become less ruminative largely remains to be seen.

STRESS AND SOCIAL SUPPORT

A key factor in reducing stress, or at least in cutting down on the effects that stress can have on the person, is social support. Social support is the term given by psychologists not only to support given through friendships and family, but also from professionals and any significant others. Generally it can come in five forms although some researchers merge some of them. The main categories are **appraisal support, emotional support, esteem support, informational support,** and **instrumental support** (Stroebe, 2000).

- **Appraisal support** is where a person is enabled or encouraged to evaluate their own state of health or problem-state, perhaps through provision of information (see below) and empowerment. They are then able to put their stressors into context.
- **Emotional support** is being loved, cared for, protected, listened to, empathised and sympathised with. It is what people often mean when they say that they have a 'shoulder to cry on'.
- **Esteem support** is a feeling that you are valued, or held in esteem, by others. Your own feelings of self-worth and self-esteem are affected by how you perceive others' opinions of you. If you feel that you are a competent and skilful person, a worthwhile person, a good person, you are more likely to be able to cope with demands put upon you, by stressors, for instance.
- **Informational support** is often provided in the first instance by a medical professional, in the case of health or illness. It is support in the form of

advice and knowledge which can assist the person in doing the right thing to look after themselves. It also takes the form of feedback, so that attending special weight loss classes where you are weighed and told the result of your efforts is, amongst other things, a form of informational support.

- **Instrumental support** is much more down-to-earth and practical. You cannot attend a weight-loss class if you have no-one to look after your children while you go, or if you have no money. If someone offers to pay for your visit, and will act as a babysitter too, then they have provided instrumental support.

A classic study of the effects of social support was reported by Berkman and Syme (1979). Thousands of people were followed over nine years in Alameda County, California. Data was obtained on social support from questions on marital status, attendance at church, contact with friends and family and membership of organisations likely to bring the person into contact with others. In addition, self-reports of various health variables and behaviours were examined, such as tobacco and alcohol intake and exercise. Basically, there was a direct relationship between amount of social support and death. Those people who received the most social support were least likely to die during the nine years, and those with least support were most likely to die. This interacted with age, such that older people with little social support were in a much more dangerous position than younger ones. This was a clear indicator that social support is directly related to health status.

The type of support available depends upon the social network of the individual, their gender, their culture, and many other factors. Ideally an individual would have all types of support available whenever they are needed, but this is probably little more than an ideal. Most people will experience problems with social support at some point, even if only because of limited resources such as money. In different cultures, friendship and family networks operate in different ways. Extended-family cultures, such as those found in India, are intuitively more likely to generate instrumental support (because more people can provide more money and equipment), and esteem and emotional support can be provided by a range of people, thus meaning that none of them feels too much strain. Of course, we often say that 'too many cooks spoil the broth', and it is also possible that a large amount of support can be overwhelming or counterproductive for some individuals. Many of us will have known people getting married who started to resent the 'help' of their families because they felt like things were being taken away from them and that people were 'interfering'. Different situations will lead to different interpretations of the support offered by the social network. Indeed, when others offer help but it is not perceived as supportive then the effects of that support are unlikely to be felt on the health of the individual and their perceived levels of stress (Dakof and Taylor, 1990).

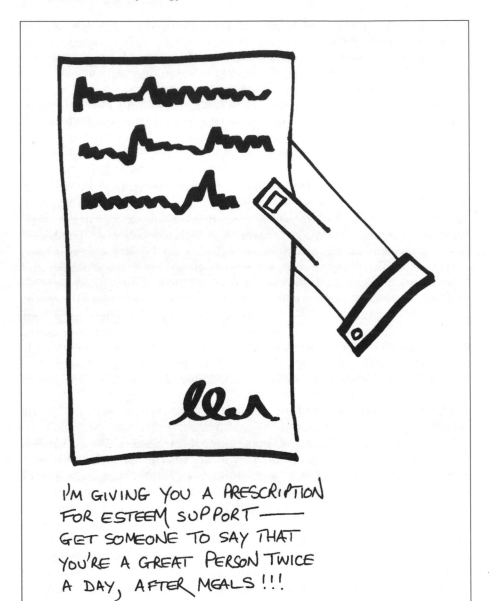

DIRECT AND BUFFERING HYPOTHESES

The effects of social support on health are seen via the stress–health link. Something occurs, so that social support prevents stress from affecting health in the way that it otherwise might. There are two ways in which this can happen: directly or indirectly.

The **direct hypothesis** is underpinned by a philosophy that social support is good for you *per se*, regardless of any stressors you are experiencing, or the powerfulness of them. The more social support you have, the better. Social support affects your mental health, this in turn affects your physical health, and therefore you are shielded directly against oncoming stressors. In effect, the absence of social support is a stressor in itself.

The **buffering hypothesis** is what the indirect path is commonly known as. Here the powerfulness of a stressor is important in determining the mediating effects of the social support. The 'buffer' of social support protects the individual against powerful stressors, but does not have much effect when the stressors are weaker. Rather than protect the person at all times, the social support they have really only works when they need it the most. This may seem rather vague, so let us take an example. In everyday life, the things which stress us are the minor hassles we have spoken of earlier: queuing in the rain for a taxi, replacement of our favourite TV programme with extended sports coverage, cutting our finger when chopping vegetables, or losing a glove on the underground. The argument is that social support is unlikely to be of much use in these circumstances. We might mention to a friend that we got wet waiting for a cab, but we are unlikely to need or ask for 'tea and sympathy' and financial or informational support! However, imagine now that a couple lose a baby due to miscarriage. Friends and family may pay them more attention, help them with getting advice from doctors, counsellors and social workers (if appropriate), or do shopping for them if they feel too upset to undertake routine activities. A family member might pay for them to have a break abroad. The couple may feel that they are in some way responsible for the loss of their baby, and those around them could provide esteem support by countering these ideas when they are expressed. As can be seen, in drastic conditions this support could make a great difference.

There is a wealth of research investigating these two hypotheses, and there is support for both. To summarise it could take up half of this book. One neat way to investigate such issues is by studying twins who have lived apart in different circumstances. They share genetic material, but backgrounds which differ can help us to discover what behaviours are attributable to that background. Kessler *et al* (1992) suggest that people differ, genetically, in the way that they find and evaluate social support. Some people may be better at finding social support, and, when support is there, they are good at perceiving the assistance as supportive. The buffering effects of social support may, therefore, be due to a person being able to make use of social support when they need it, that is in times of great stress. At other times, they don't need it, so it is not going to show up as a buffer. Equally, certain people may be good at *creating* a social support network when they need it. If they don't need it, during minor hassles, they don't set it up, and so it can hardly act as a buffer!

Of course, not all people have the gift of drawing upon individuals and organisations effectively and efficiently when required. They are, perhaps, the people who most need skills training to alleviate their stress.

STRESS AND CONTROL

The links between personal control, perceived or actual, and health have been studied by health psychologists interested in stress. Control is essentially the extent to which a person feels that they are able to make a difference to things around them and to their own life circumstances and health. Helplessness might, therefore, be argued to be the extreme opposite of control. We deal with control elsewhere in this book, in the form of LoC, for instance.

One of the most common areas of study for the link between health, stress and control is the realm of work. People are often stressed by work, and they are equally often lacking control over the nature of the work. After all, it is rare that someone can do more or less what they like at work. Someone else usually controls the work done, the way that it is done, and the product is assessed and verified. The very phrase 'quality control' gives away the sense in which work is usually directed by other people. Someone produces, someone else controls for the quality of what is produced, often by creating more and more rules for people to work by. Frankenhaeuser (1975) examined control and stress in a sample of sawmill workers in Sweden. Many such workers have remarkably monotonous jobs, repeating the same prescribed action over and over again, day after day, for often a whole working life. The work can be as unvaried as cutting a piece of wood to a set size, then another, then another, and so on. Frankenhaeuser measured the biochemical effects of stress, finding that the sawmill workers had high levels of catecholamines, associated with stress. They also reported more than average signs of stress such as hypertension, headaches and digestive tract problems. The key fact here is that the workers do not choose what size the wood must be cut to; that is done for them. They do not have any say in anything that they do, and so feel like their work is entirely out of their control. For most people, this can be a demoralising process which affects stress levels and, hence, health. Of course, we must not forget that there are probably people for whom control itself is stressful. Not everyone wants responsibility. In fact, the evidence shows that too much control can also be a bad thing. Other typically high-stress occupations include management and medicine, law and teaching. Here people often have high degrees of autonomy. The stress in these occupations is often attributable to the pressure that being responsible creates. Being the person who can be blamed when things go wrong, the person who makes decisions, is just as stressful as never having a say.

HARDINESS

Hardiness is a concept first put forward by Kobasa (1979) which describes a set of traits which can protect a person from the effects of stress, and which includes control as a factor. This is a personality-based approach which focuses on characteristics of the individual rather than of the environment (contrasted, therefore, with social support). A 'hardy' person copes well with stress. They are, according to Kobasa, a person who has a high sense of personal control (that is, someone who believes that they can *do* things about their life and health), a person who is committed to things, and a person who likes challenges, and sees them as a good thing in life. The hardy person views change as a positive, rather than a negative, thing. Of course, you may remember earlier that a person who does this is, if you look at it in a different way, employing a positive reappraisal coping strategy. In respect to commitment, the committed person values and finds purpose in their work and their social contacts. A hardy person is often a resilient individual, the type of person about whom people say 'she can cope with anything'. They are the survivors of this world, the people who seem to 'take whatever is thrown at them'. They are the people who 'bounce back'.

Hardiness is generally measured using a combination of scales measuring each of the individual components of reaction to change, control, and commitment. For instance, control can be indexed by an LoC measure. There is a moderate amount of evidence to show that hardiness acts as a buffer against stress, although the evidence is countered by studies showing little effect of hardiness, as defined by Kobasa, on reactions to stress.

One problem with hardiness is that the factors which comprise it are not always found together in the same person. They do not correlate very highly with each other. They should, of course, if hardiness can be seen as *one* collective thing. The counter argument could be that hardy individuals are those people in whom high levels of these three factors *are* found.

WOMEN AND STRESS

Health psychologists have been guilty, over the years, of concentrating on a male-oriented view of stress and its effects (Carroll and Niven, 1993). Since men are most at risk from heart disease, at least until women 'catch up' after the menopause, reducing stress, and therefore heart disease, was seen as something that should be done mainly for men. However, women do suffer heart disease, but also the range of other problems which affect men when they are under stress: bowel problems, headaches, skin disorders and so on.

There is evidence that men and women differ in their reactions to stress, and in their general levels of perceived stress. Of course, most societies treat men and women differently, and so it is a moot point as to whether these differences inhere in the social and cultural variation between the sexes or in the biological. In an important early paper, Waldron (1976) argues that women live longer than men because men often cope with stress in ways which are harmful, such as the smoking of cigarettes and excess drinking of alcohol. You may, however, be aware that the incidence of smoking in females is increasing whilst in men it is not, and that a pattern of drinking behaviour similar to that of men is starting to surface in young women. Whether this will remain a gender-biased coping strategy in just a few years time is looking doubtful.

Whilst there are inequalities based upon gender, such as there are in health, education, employment and most areas of life, women may experience a similar lack of control over their lives as did the Swedish sawmill workers referred to earlier. Since stress can be a result of lack of control, women are clear candidates for high levels of stress (and they do, indeed, report higher levels than men, according to Carroll and Niven, 1993). However, since their age of death is consistently and significantly higher than men, they may perhaps be coping with stressors in a more effective way.

Using the distinction between ruminators and non-ruminators mentioned earlier, Strauss et al (1997) compared male and female responses to depression in undergraduate students, using a self-report questionnaire. They found that, in general, men tended to use distraction (i.e. non-rumination) as a coping mechanism and women tended to be greater ruminators, but in a further study they discovered that this pattern was less clear, with women ruminating more than men but with men and women equally likely to report using distraction. The authors warn that self-report measures may lead to distortions of the facts since the stereotype that men do not ruminate may influence their reports of rumination.

Hyyppae et al (1988) studied gender differences in biochemical responses to distress, alongside their psychological and other characteristics. Twenty-five female and 34 male patients were investigated on admission to hospital with low back pain and five years later after treatment. Cortisol is a hormone related to pain and stress experience. They measured blood concentrations of this hormone, and found that on admission to hospital there was a major sex difference in levels, but that after treatment other psychological factors predicted it too. They conclude that the body's chemical reaction to stress and pain can be moderated by factors such as coping strategy, which is gender-related. Therefore, by modifying their behaviours, men and women can achieve better coping not just psychologically but physically.

REDUCING STRESS

In addition to the very real and significant ways in which social support can moderate stress, there are literally thousands of ways to reduce stress available to people, either free-of-charge or by paying individuals or organisations for either knowledge or equipment to facilitate relaxation. Some of these are more unusual and 'wacky' than others, but most can be classified into the ways in which they effect their stress relief.

Exercise is one way to relieve stress. Studies have shown a relationship between the ability of the body to cope with stress and indulgence in exercise, especially aerobic exercise. Sinyor *et al* (1983) compared people who exercise regularly with those who do not in their hormonal reactions to an artificial stressor. They found that the exercisers had better rates of recovery from the stress.

Relaxation is another path to reducing stress, achieved commonly through things such as meditation. In Japanese offices, workers are often encouraged to exercise at work, and calming sounds such as that of rain are played through the company public address system. Reducing stress, therefore, is not just a private, individual thing: it can be a public or group activity. In China, early morning tai chi sessions are to be seen in open-air, public squares. Scientific involvement in relaxation-based stress reduction has, at times, centred around the issue of biofeedback. Biofeedback concerns the process of wiring up a person to measure their vital signs such as heart rate and blood pressure, and enabling them to monitor them with a view to changing them consciously, at will. The idea is that by learning to lower blood pressure or heart rate, the individual can relax more effectively and take control over bodily functions which have a central role in health. The problem is that reducing stress signs during periods of non-stress does not necessarily generalise to times when stressors are present (Holmes, 1984).

Time management is a common technique aimed at reducing stress indirectly, by eliminating the feelings of being under time-pressures. In the business world there are expert consultants in time management who can demand high fees for teaching people how to manage their time effectively. Companies realise that an employee who manages their time well is one who not only gets more work done in the time available, but who is also less stressed. Less stress equates directly to better health, and this means fewer days off work. Stress is estimated to result in millions of lost days of work per year in most developed countries. Aside from the official statistics on this, there are also the unofficial cases. When some people pretend to be physically ill because they cannot face going in to work, it is likely to be stress which is putting them into that position.

Time management can be achieved relatively easily, if you have the time for it! Indeed, many people fail to manage time effectively because they fail to find time to set about managing time. Time management techniques can be picked up from little books at a small cost, or someone can invest in very expensive, individually tailored programmes from a 'personal trainer'. Either way, well managed time can mean a healthy person.

Social support enhancement is a key factor in cutting down on the damaging effects of stress. It is not always easy to do, simply because it is often painfully difficult for people to make friends. However, by joining clubs and 'getting out more' people who are lonely may find ways to generate more social support, which as we have seen can have a significant impact on their health, even their likely age of death. Additionally, TV campaigns such as those in the United Kingdom, asking people to check on their neighbours regularly, especially if they are old and live alone, may assist in this. The purpose of such a request goes beyond personal safety, and can easily contribute to psychological health.

Control enhancement is another issue which is achieved by a range of techniques. We have already identified that stress is something that can be moderated by perceived control over situations. By effectively tampering with perceived control, we can make a difference to perceived stress. How can we achieve this? Firstly, control can be increased in real terms, by people's employers, for instance, changing the nature of work to allow for employees to make decisions and to control their working practices within reason. Secondly, cognitive–behavioural techniques are a good way, involving changing people's perceptions of themselves and their sense of control. By a range of methods, usually involving some kind of more or less sophisticated conditioning, people learn to think differently.

Stress inoculation training (Meichenbaum and Deffenbacher, 1988) is a specific form of stress management. It involves training people in new skills, through three phases: conceptualization, skills acquisition and rehearsal, and application. In the conceptualization phase, people are taught what the body does as a reaction to stress, and what the common psychological consequences are. They are made to analyse their own reactions to stress. In the skills acquisition and rehearsal phase, people are asked to try out alternative reactions. So instead of waiting in a queue provoking the usual thoughts of 'Come on, come on, hurry up, come on, I haven't got all day . . .', the person is encouraged to think something like 'Keep calm . . . the queue will go down in time . . . my anxiousness will not make a difference to the queue.' They are taught techniques of stress reduction such as relaxation, and positive coping styles are emphasised. In the application phase, people have to really try these things out in their lives, keeping records to see the differences they make to them. This is, in essence, an extended form of cognitive–behavioural therapy, which has been shown to have a moderate degree of success in helping stressed individuals.

STRESS IN HEALTH PROFESSIONALS

The health professions, like many others, are high-stress occupations. Doctors and nurses commonly work long hours, and have some particularly difficult problems to deal with. In careers of this type, people often report that they are unable to 'switch off' from work at the end of a shift. Their work remains on their minds, especially when during the day they have been witness to deaths and to the aftermath of horrific accidents. Chronic stress in those professions which have a high level of contact with clients (teaching, law, policing, medicine and the like) can have some particularly strange effects on the person, the constellation of which has been termed **burnout**.

Burnout is quite separate from stress, and is really best seen as a result of stress rather than a form of it. The term was coined by Freudenberger (1974), and has since been used extensively to describe the physical and emotional changes which can occur when job stress forces an individual to adapt to their environment (Maslach, 1982). Long-term work stress can create a situation where people turn to alcohol or other drugs in order to cope, develop many physical symptoms of stress, and begin to lose interest in things around them. They also, typically, start to lack sympathy for people in their environment. Losing a sense of caring for one's clients is, of course, particularly damaging when one is working in a so-called caring profession. No-one would wish to be treated by a nurse who simply does not care. In many ways emotional flatness which occurs in burnout can be considered to be a biological, protective reaction which has become exaggerated. It can be seen as a way of turning off from the outside world to protect the individual. However, it is usually also damaging to them, and can be considerably disturbing: for example, they are usually distressed when they realise that they seem to have stopped caring about people and what happens to them. The three main characteristics of burnout, according to Maslach (1982) are *depersonalisation*, as described above, *emotional exhaustion* (where the person feels simply tired of things, and unable to muster up the resources to be an emotional being) and *perceived inadequacy* (where the person feels that they are losing their ability to do their job properly).

It is not difficult to imagine how a doctor experiencing burnout will treat their patients. Lacking energy, lacking empathy or sympathy, and lacking self-confidence, they will neither care much about what happens to them, nor believe that they are likely to be able to make a difference to them. In the best case, the patient receives no help, in the worst the patient is harmed (by, for example, a doctor who takes less care in administering an injection and so damages tissue, or does not doublecheck a drug dosage and ends up poisoning the patient).

Hillhouse and Adler (1996) looked at burnout in nurses. They analysed the results from questionnaires completed by 297 hospital nurses, and challenged the notion that burnout is simply the result of work stress. They found that burnout acted as an intervening variable *between* work stress and physical/emotional symptoms. What this means is that individuals experiencing work stress may not always burn out, but can bypass that stage and experience physical and affective (emotional) symptoms directly. However, when burnout occurs it is a distinct phenomenon which occurs before the main physical and mental signs of stress. Treating burnout is not going to be effective unless the reasons for its occurrence are treated. This means, of course, that working conditions must be changed if burnout is not to occur. Research seems to indicate that burnout is most likely to occur when the degree of contact with patients is high. Doctors who spend a larger proportion of their time in non-clinical activities (teaching, attending conferences, administration) are less likely to report feelings of depersonalization and emotional apathy. Therefore, a good balance between these activities is probably the healthiest option for most physicians and nurses. In some cases, a change is as good as a rest.

Case In Point: Greg

Greg is a 40-year old car designer, who was made redundant some time ago. When this happened, he did not tell his partner, and instead looked for work during the three months his contract still had to run. Rather than worry other people, he carried on as usual, but spent his lunch hour on the internet seeking work. Sadly, he did not find work in that time. Losing his job and failing to find another left him feeling useless. He decided not to tell his partner, and to continue leaving the house every morning as if for work and returning at the end of the day. During the day, he looked for work. He did not find it easy to lie in this way, but did not find it easy to tell his partner the truth. He began to drink a little more heavily than usual, because he would go to a bar at lunchtime. He felt guilty spending money on alcohol in this way, which meant that he would often walk the six miles home.

As the weeks went by he became more and more concerned that he was not finding work. At this point he confided in Tony, his best friend, who was shocked at the news. Tony offered to lend him money to 'tide him over' at this difficult time, but Greg refused, anxious that he did not end up in debt to anyone.

Greg began to develop headaches, which at first he put down to alcohol at lunchtime. Eventually, they were bad enough that he had to stay away from 'work'. His partner, being kind, rang his ex-employer to let them know that he would not be there one particular morning, and that was when the truth came out. An argument ensued, and Greg left the house in a temper. Not knowing what to do or to whom to turn for help, Greg rang Tony at work, who offered to put him up for a few days until things calmed down.

Commentary

Greg, it seems from this, shows a mixture of coping styles. Whilst there is distance coping (carrying on as normal), there is escape–avoidance coping (alcohol) and there is also some planful problem solving, in that he is trying to find work. He actively avoids seeking social support, and turns down Tony's first offer of instrumental support (money). However, he succumbs to his second offer of instrumental support (temporary accommodation).

Greg demonstrates cognitive dissonance when he feels guilty about lying but equally distressed at the prospect of having to tell his partner the truth. Cognitive dissonance often prevents people from acting in an appropriate way, because, like Greg, they may tend to choose the option that involves least action, even if it does have moral implications (i.e. he prefers to lie than to deal with the stress of telling his partner). This is also an example of avoidant behaviour, as opposed to approach coping.

The signs of stress begin to show (headaches) but Greg seeks an alternative explanation, either because he does not recognise headaches as a sign of stress or because he does but prefers to re-label them. This re-labelling might be a type of denial.

Given what we have seen so far, a solution to Greg's problem might be difficult to find, simply because he is not a textbook case, even though he is a case in a textbook! He shows, like many real people, a blend of feelings, many of which do not sit easily together. Some social support is acceptable to him, but some isn't. He prefers to be secretive than open, it seems, which means that seeking help might be difficult for him. If he finds work, the problems may disappear immediately, but if he does not, he needs a more suitable way of coping with stress than alcohol. It does not seem, from the details here, that Greg will seek help from professionals, such as counsellors. Therefore, the best way forward is if Greg talks the problems through with Tony. Provided that this happens, and that Tony is able to offer good advice and some emotional and esteem support (since Greg feels useless), Greg may be able to make plans to confront his unemployment, and his partner, and to find a way of co-operating with his partner who may support him further.

The purpose of this case study is to demonstrate that Greg cannot be simply given advice by a professional, which will then be exactly matched to his needs. People have to *seek* advice and support. If they do not, we cannot identify that they need it, and it would be unethical to thrust support onto someone who did not request it. In addition, given Greg's situation and his blend of coping styles, help for him would not be simple. He is not unusual. His complexity is what characterises most human beings. This is why health psychologists, and all health professionals, have a difficult job to do.

CONCLUDING REMARKS

This chapter has brushed the surface of the research into stress. Nothing else could be done in a volume of this size. If you take one message away from reading this, let it be that stress is complicated, like other things psychologists study, and that it depends on factors both intrinsic and extrinsic to the individual. Stress is a problem for us all. Most of us are likely to experience it, many to debilitating degrees. It is a problem for health psychologists in particular. It represents one of the more easily demonstrable cases of a link between the body and the mind, and as such it is something that a professional health psychologist needs to be able to do something about. In some ways, as we learn more about stress, combating it becomes more difficult. Not only does it become more complicated, but the world keeps on changing. A consequence of the type of world we increasingly live in is higher levels of perceived stress. For every time-saving device comes a new stressor. Computers are great because they do things quickly, but we rant and rave when they crash. Mobile telephones can save lives, time and trouble, but also create stress if we are worried that they might cause ill health, or when we would rather be incommunicado in order to have time to ourselves. We keep on finding new ways to become stressed. We are, therefore, unlikely to eliminate stress for good.

Study questions

1. How do *you* cope with stress? Does it work?

2. Is stress an unavoidable consequence of being human?

FURTHER READING

Calnan, M., Wainwright, D., Forsythe, M., Wall, B. and Almond, S. (2001): Mental health and stress in the workplace: the case of general practice in the UK. *Social Science and Medicine*, **52**, 499–507.

A startling paper, identifying that almost a quarter of staff in general practice are suffering from mental distress.

Cassidy, T. (1999): *Stress, Cognition and Health*. London: Routledge.

A short, readable introduction to the relationship between stress, health and our thoughts and feelings.

6

The Appetites

INTRODUCTION

Appetites of one sort or another often drive people to behave the way that they do. We crave certain things, and we will often go to considerable lengths to satisfy our appetites. There are some appetites which are fundamental to our existence, such as the desire to eat and drink or engage in sexual intercourse, which we can view as being instinctual. Without food and drink, we die. Without sexual intercourse, there is no propagation of animal species. It makes sense that over millions of years of evolution we have developed an overriding requirement to feed ourselves, and, for most people, to want to have sex and to raise children. There are also more 'sophisticated' appetites which are more artificial, and are, largely, a product of modern ways of life. These include the desire to consume or use drugs such as nicotine in the form of cigarettes, alcohol, and substances such as marijuana, cocaine or heroin. These latter appetites cannot be seen as instinctual, for what should be obvious reasons. We do not even need to become addicted to food, because we have an intrinsic requirement for it. In the case of tobacco, alcohol, and other drugs, the abuses rely on the fact that the substances themselves are often physically and/or psychologically addictive.

In this chapter, research into the main appetitive behaviours is described. In health psychology, there has been more emphasis on some of these than others, something which will become apparent as the chapter unfolds. Three major areas of interest for health psychologists, but also for doctors, and for clinical psychologists and health educators and promotors, have been sexual health, smoking and alcohol-related behaviour. In addition, the study of disorders of eating has been undertaken.

EATING DISORDERS

To many people, the term 'eating disorder' generates thoughts and images of people with anorexia nervosa, i.e. those people who avoid eating because they seek a slimmer body until they seriously damage their health. However, any problem of eating is really an eating disorder. Therefore, it includes all extremes of eating behaviour, from people who eat too much and become obese, to people who eat virtually nothing at all, and including those people who eat poor diets with preponderances of certain items, and even including those rare individuals who are 'addicted' to eating non-foodstuffs such as clay or paper. Virtually no psychological research has been directed towards this latter category, and so this will not be dealt with here, but it is important that the reader is at least aware of this unusual type of eating disorder. It is, perhaps, an area for future investigation.

Eating too much

Many societies around the world face a growing problem of obesity. As many as 14% of people in England (Seidell and Rissenen, 1998) are clinically overweight, to a degree that doctors believe can be damaging to health in the long term. A heavier society is one which relies more upon health services, which costs more money. Naturally, then, there is a significant incentive for governments and health authorities to try to create slimmer, healthier nations. Bear in mind, however, that to suggest that obese people should be slimmer *for any reason other than health* is not acceptable. Researchers in obesity tread a fine line between promoting health issues and promulgating ideas that being overweight is unattractive and socially undesirable. Cosmetic dieting is another issue entirely, and one that health researchers are probably best served by avoiding.

The consequences of chronic obesity are well documented. People who are highly overweight have an increased risk of heart disease, because they put strain on their heart by having to move around a heavier body, but also because the heart builds up fatty deposits around it which cause the organ to have to work harder. Equally, the kind of diet which encourages weight gain is generally high in fat. High-fat diets cause plaques of fat to build up in the arteries, clogging them, something known as atheroma. Overweight people have a greater likelihood of developing diabetes mellitus. They tend to live less long than people of statistically normal weight. They may have reduced self-image, which can lead to a loss of self-esteem (Miller and Downey, 1999). In this research, 71 studies of self-esteem measures and body weight were synthesised to show that the relationship between these factors was significant, and larger for women than for men. However, although statistically significant, the correlation is still relatively modest. There is certainly no obvious and direct 'gain weight – lose self-esteem' link. Foster *et al* (1996) looked at depression in people over time and established that weight gains and losses were not associated with depressive episodes and remissions from depression, contradicting the view that people who gain weight feel sad as a result. The problem with this type of research is that it overlooks individual differences in eating and emotional behaviour. Some people will not feel happy or sad in relation to their body shape or size. However, of those that do some will, perhaps, become more depressed as a result of gaining weight, whereas others might gain weight as a result of depression by some other cause (so-called 'comfort eating'). The various time lags between eating behaviour and emotional reactions to weight gain and other life-events may mean that there is no discernible relationship between body mass and depression when groups of people rather than individuals are looked at. In addition, such studies tend to use tools to measure depression at clinical levels. Sub-clinical depression is more difficult to quantify, but this is where body image might affect the obese person more. Becoming overweight might not make people clinically depressed, with all its concomitant symptoms of changes in sleeping patterns, sociability, dietary habits, interest in life in general, and so on, but it might simply make them feel a little more sad or unhappy. Currently we are less able to measure these small effects than we are full-scale depression.

Why do people overeat? Why is it so difficult to lose weight and then to maintain a healthy proportion of body fat? The first question is likely to have hundreds of answers, and psychologists are only beginning to provide some of them, after many years of research. People may overeat, or at least may be overweight, because their culture and values tend to expect it. In Tonga, a very large proportion of people are overweight by Western standards and having excess body fat is the norm for both men and women. In some cultures, specifically those around and including India, being moderately overweight is perceived as a sign of riches, and in a man it is indicative, it is believed by some, of the fact that his wife is looking after him well. The meaning of 'being overweight' is, therefore, different around the world, and throughout time as values change. People may overeat because their bodies are constructed that way, either because their brains are 'set' that way or because they have more fat cells or a different metabolism. People may overeat to provide comfort and reduce stress or boredom. People with a full social life, or a career where entertaining business clients is part of the job, may find themselves eating more because they have to go out to dinner and eat rich food more often.

Whilst there is by no means a consistent and clear relationship between energy intake, energy expenditure and body fat, the human body cannot maintain its weight unless a certain intake of energy is guaranteed. The metabolic processes of the body adjust themselves to trends in food consumption and exercise behaviour, but generally a person eating too little will lose weight in the longer term and a person eating too much will gain it. The view that some people seem to gain weight no matter how much they control their eating or, more prevalent, that some people cannot gain weight no matter how much they eat, is partly borne out by research. A review of 29 studies on food intake by obese people did not show that overweight people ate more than people of normal weight (Spitzer and Rodin, 1981), however, the question we must ask is how much the overweight people are supposed to eat to maintain a normal bodyweight. It is quite possible that they are eating too much *for them*. The metabolic rates of individuals can have dramatic effects on body size. The body acts like an engine, using up fuel to convert it into kinetic (movement) energy. The way that an engine is configured to combust fuel can mean that, compared to a similar engine, it produces more movement per unit of fuel burned. In theory, two different bodies can require vastly different amounts of energy intake to do the same work. People differ in so many ways. A person with a relatively fast and powerful heartbeat, for instance, may require more energy to maintain their heart's activity than a person with a relatively slow, weak one. Over days and weeks of activity, this might add up to a considerable difference in energy requirements. Some people are generally more physically active than others, not just in obvious ways, such as in how much sport they engage in or what their work involves, but also in more subtle ways, such as how much they might thrash around in their sleep, or how much they talk in an average day, or how tense their muscles are in their basic resting state. If a person has slightly more tense muscles than another, this might mean that their body requires a little more energy, even in its most relaxed state. Multiply this effect over years, and the difference in food consumed as a result might again be significant.

Most attempts by psychologists and overweight individuals to modify eating behaviour and thus achieve and maintain a normal body weight ultimately fail (Garner and Wooley, 1991). Those people who manage to lose weight commonly start to gain weight again once the restrictive diet is complete. The problem is that being overweight can be such a health problem it is simply not possible to give up trying to find ways to reduce the body fat of certain people. The lack of significant success over many years is not a reason to relinquish the endeavour. Since it is so difficult to change the eating habits, and thus bodyweights, of obese people, many health researchers have concentrated their efforts on preventing people becoming obese in the first place. What is clear is that preventing children from becoming obese needs to involve the family, since poor eating habits could be learned at home. However, since there seems to be a strong genetic basis for obesity, with identical twins showing more similarities in weight than non-identical twins (Allison *et al*, 1994), even the attempt to prevent children gaining weight might be associated with great difficulties. If we are fighting against nature, as it were, nature is quite likely to win. Overcoming millions of years of evolution is not something that a few thousand psychologists can do that easily.

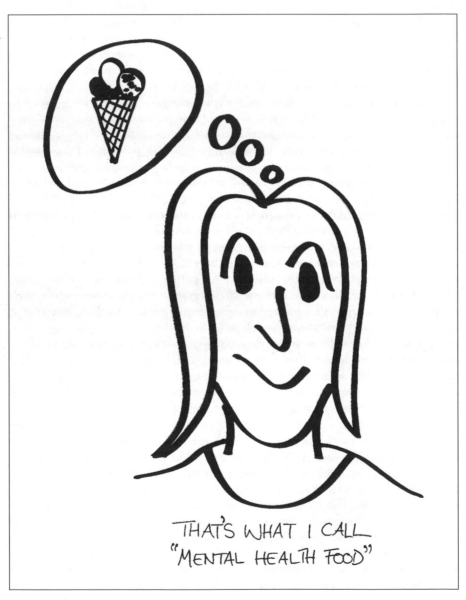

Some researchers argue that there is a natural **set-point** of bodyweight, which bodily mechanisms, particularly the hypothalamus, strive to achieve (Keesey, 1980). Sometimes the set-point can be underweight, sometimes overweight, compared to the average person. When a person undereats *for them*, their body adjusts, creating cravings for food and slowing down the metabolism to use up less energy. When a person overeats *for them*, their body reacts by increasing metabolic rate and making the person feel less like eating. In addition, there is also some evidence that obese and non-obese individuals differ in the number of fat cells (adipocytes) that they possess (Sjöström, 1980). So, not only do obese people have more fat stored in each fat cell but they have more fat cells available to fill. There is even a belief amongst tissue scientists that once fat cells are formed, they are never lost. Again, this is another obstacle in our path to reducing ill health due to obesity.

A seminal work on personality types and overeating comes from Herman and Mack (1975). They categorised people into **restrained** and **unrestrained** eaters. Restrained eaters are constantly conscious about what they eat and are careful to avoid certain foods. They may be frequently on calorie-controlled diets, and for them the business of eating can be a fraught one. They are the people who may report feeling 'guilty' after having the occasional chocolate bar, or who will, perhaps, miss a meal in order to make up for an additional slice of toast at breakfast. In contrast to this, the unrestrained eaters are people who simply eat what they like, when they like. They do not tend to count calories. You would be forgiven for thinking that unrestrained eaters are the people who become obese, but the relationship is far from being that simple. In fact, many theorists believe that unrestrained eating can be quite healthy and is nothing more than a form of 'listening' to the body's needs and supplying them by giving in to cravings and hunger. Restrained eaters, on the other hand, interfere with the body's natural processes by trying to alter and change their dietary habits. They develop eating habits which are often unhealthy, and are more likely to engage in bouts of 'disinhibition'. This is where their usual strictness and care gives way to abandonment and bingeing. Restrained eaters typically feel dejected when they 'break the rules' of a diet or spoil an eating plan, and as a result break the rules even more. They are more likely to say something like: 'I've eaten one slice of cake, so I might as well have another because the damage is done.' Not only this, but these people will often, as a result of showing a lack of 'willpower', develop lower levels of self-esteem. This may then be implicated in further bouts of overeating. Evidence that restraint leads to overeating comes from Wardle and Beales (1988). They took obese women and split them between three conditions; in one they were expected to engage in a low-calorie diet, another group was engaged in exercise, and a further group was simply enrolled into the study but given no instructions either to exercise or to diet. After a number of weeks, measures of food intake indicated that the women in the dieting condition actually ate more than the others.

One difficulty with the restrained/unrestrained dichotomy is that it can imply that people are either a restrained or an unrestrained eater. Some people, however, may experience periods of one type of behaviour followed by periods of the other and back again. Some people may be at a point on a continuum between restrained and unrestrained eating habits, rather than in one 'camp' or another. Another problem is that this theory would predict that people who restrain themselves will succumb to periods of bingeing. It cannot, therefore, explain how people with anorexia nervosa can starve themselves to the point of death and avoid food completely, with no sign of any craving for food. In the next section, we look at this phenomenon.

Eating too little

Just as being overweight is injurious to health, so is being underweight. In fact, death can occur at either end of the spectrum of body weights. When a person cannot eat because of a famine, or refuses to eat, the body tries other ways to survive. When fat reserves are depleted, and no external food source is available, the body starts working on other tissues, principally muscle, which is a good source of calories (steak, chicken breast and fillet of fish are simply animal muscle). The body starts to derive energy from burning up muscle tissue, and so the body literally eats itself up. Women who eat too little start to notice bodily warning signs, perhaps before men who do. A woman whose body fat falls below healthy levels will stop menstruating (Clare, 1998). After all, the need to stay alive overrides the drive to reproduce in most species. **Anorexia nervosa** (AN) is an illness characterised by an intense desire to lose weight. (Please do not confuse anorexia nervosa with anorexia; the latter simply means 'loss of appetite' and is quite normal in many illnesses. Most of us have experienced anorexia at some time in our lives, but far fewer of us anorexia nervosa.) The vast majority of people who develop AN are female, and below the age of 30; the average age of onset is 16–17 years (Clare, 1998). By definition, AN is a mental illness, since it is entirely the perceptions of the person which determine their desire to lose weight. A person with AN commonly believes that they are 'too fat', even when they are thin to the point where their bodies are suffering as a result and it is obvious to the casual observer that they are genuinely underweight. There is a characteristic attitude to the possibility of being fat that is best described as a real fear, rather than simply a negative view of it. Some people with AN simply fail to see that they are underweight; others do recognise it, but become fixated on the belief that their body is mis-shapen because one or more parts of it are carrying too much weight. Rather than see their whole body as overweight, some people with AN see their body as generally underweight, but with overweight buttocks, or calves, or abdomen. Thus, in these people, the desire to have a flat stomach may mean that the rest of the body becomes dangerously thin. People with AN achieve their underweight state by one of three means; reducing energy intake by dieting or starvation, increasing energy consumption by exercising, or purging the body of nutrients by using emetics or laxatives. Any or all of these may be followed to extremes where death occurs. Self-worth tends to be strongly associated with body image, such that a person with AN is quite likely to believe that they are an unpopular and generally worthless person if they are overweight, and that by losing weight they will gain self-esteem, and the esteem of others.

Research into AN has demonstrated that it has a familial component and so may have a genetic basis. It is more common in women of middle- and upper-middle-class origins than in working-class women, suggesting social influences, and it is more prevalent in women involved in the performing arts and in sport, probably because of the perceived need for a slim physique in these professions (French and Jeffery, 1994). Psychological research into AN, especially within health psychology itself, is much rarer than into some illnesses. Principally, AN and other eating disorders are of greater research interest to clinical psychologists, since they are the people who have most contact with people who are ill because of AN.

Other disturbances of eating

Another illness which is psychological in origin and also hinges around eating behaviour and body and self-image is **bulimia nervosa** (BN). This is similar to AN, but individuals follow a cyclical pattern of behaviour, bingeing and purging in succession. A person with BN may consume a day's calories or more at a single sitting, filling themselves until they are sick. The purging rarely works when it is an attempt to lose weight, and so, unlike people with AN, bulimics often maintain their bodyweight, which can be above average for their height but not necessarily in the category of obesity (many BN sufferers, however, are normal weight). Therefore, people with BN do not tend to achieve what they wish to achieve. This makes it different from AN in that the methods used by AN sufferers to lose weight do work, even if to extreme degrees. BN tends to be found in the same types of people as AN, that is mainly young women. Another difference between AN and BN is self-awareness and accuracy of perception. Whilst people with AN may perceive themselves as thin and continue to diet, people with BN are often in tune with their body size to a greater degree. They are also more likely to be aware that their eating habits are unhealthy and are damaging to them, but are almost 'addicted' to the binge–purge cycle. This awareness that things are wrong can lead to depression. The physical act of purging can produce digestive and cardiovascular problems. The cluster of health issues can sometimes, therefore, prove too much for a person with an eating disorder. Suicide is not uncommon in bulimic individuals.

One of the first health professionals to notice signs of either anorexia or bulimia nervosa is a dentist (Robb and Smith, 1996). Repeated vomiting causes dental erosion, partly because of the corrosive nature of digestive fluids. Therefore, diagnostic clues can come from a variety of sources, and a good referral mechanism between health professionals is essential.

A further disorder is **binge eating disorder** (BED). This is like BN but without the episodes of purging. Therefore, people with BED are more likely to be obese because they eat large quantities but do not engage in behaviours intended to compensate for their bingeing. BED is more common than either AN or BN. This might be because it represents an extreme form of a behaviour pattern that many people display from time to time. Most of us on occasion have eaten quite a lot more than we should, and expressed it perhaps in phrases like 'I really pigged out'. Doing this too often is essentially BED. We should dwell for a moment on phrases like 'pigging out'. They, perhaps, reflect the negative attitudes we tend to hold in Western societies towards eating large amounts and becoming fat. In essence, we are comparing obese people to animals; and not even animals which we tend to have much respect for. Such attitudes may be partly to blame for the existence of eating disorders.

Nutritional imbalances and dietary toxins

Healthy eating, by definition, makes people need doctors less often. There are probably billions of people in the world who could benefit from a better diet. These billions are not at risk from immediate disease or illness as a result of their eating habits, but may be setting themselves up for future health problems. Eating fried potatoes every day is unlikely to cause health problems in the short-term. But after 30 years of this, perhaps combined with other dietary idiosyncrasies such as avoiding fresh fruit or drinking a lot of coffee, a person could find themselves with heart disease. By educating people about healthy diets and promoting good eating habits, doctors can hope to make their work easier in the future. (Of course, not all people have a wide choice in what they eat: poverty or geographical location can restrict diet, as can individual allergies to foodstuffs.)

Chemicals in our food, either ones which are there naturally or ones which are there in processed food to add flavour or colour or to preserve food, are often implicated in health problems. There is some highly debated evidence to suggest, for instance, that behavioural problems in children can be traced back to food additives.

Caffeine is a common drug which has some strong effects on the nervous system. It is an addictive substance, which causes increased alertness but can also damage the cardiovascular system if abused. It is present in coffee, tea, cola drinks and chocolate. Even decaffeinated tea and coffee often contain other related chemicals with similar effects; removing caffeine does not always remove other theobromines and theophyllines. The vast amount of tea and coffee consumed throughout the world is indirect evidence of their addictive properties. Caffeine can increase blood pressure, although it seems that serious consequences for the functioning of the heart are only likely when the intake of caffeine is very great. In a meta-analysis of many studies on coffee consumption, Kawachi, Colditz and Stone (1994) found that there were no significant effects of caffeine on incidence of heart disease.

SMOKING

In Britain, in 1996, just under 30% of people smoked (Office of National Statistics, 1999). The effects of smoking, and of passive smoking (ingesting other people's cigarette smoke from the air) are probably well known to the reader. You probably know that there is a relationship between smoking and lung disease such as lung cancer, for instance. Ask yourself how you know that. The answer is, partly, because health education and health promotion campaigns can really work. Since the research into smoking first began to show that it is associated with health problems, health professionals around the world have been trying to get this message across to people. Even if you smoke, you are highly likely to be aware of the risks you are taking, especially since health warnings are printed on cigarette packets in most countries, if not all. When a campaign is at its most successful, the media tend to take up part of the campaign too. Most of us will, at some point in our lives, have seen or heard a documentary programme on TV or radio about the tobacco industry or about the health issues around smoking. Many TV companies have strict rules about showing people smoking on TV, and cigarette advertising on television is not allowed in Britain.

Of course, given that the anti-smoking ethos is so strongly supported in many countries, we must ask why so many people still smoke, and why so many young people take up the habit of smoking. Fifty or more years ago, people did not really know that smoking could be harmful. Now that most people do, why do they still do it?

We cannot deal here with every explanation of smoking that has ever been put forward in the history of psychology, since, for example, psychoanalytic theories first purported that smoking was a form of fixation with oral activity. There are entire books on psychological aspects of smoking. Instead, we focus on a selection of explanations.

The content of tobacco cannot be ignored, since there is a strongly addictive element present: nicotine. Like any addictive substance, once people become used to having nicotine in their blood they crave it when it is absent, or when the levels fall too low. This view is known as the **nicotine-regulation model**, and was developed by Schachter (1977). However, this fails to account for why people begin smoking in the first place, or why some people smoke (albeit small amounts) even though they do not seem to be addicted in any measurable, physical sense. We call such smokers 'chippers' (Shiffman *et al*, 1995). It is, therefore, important to look at psychological factors, especially prior to addiction itself having begun.

It is likely that a combination of social, cultural, environmental and biological factors are involved in both up-take and maintenance of the habit of smoking. Most smokers begin the habit in their teenage years, a time when people are impressionable and open to significant peer pressure. Killen *et al* (1997) have shown that having friends who smoke is significantly related to the odds of a person experimenting with smoking, such that the more friends a person has the greater the chance that they too will try cigarettes. Once a person has tried cigarettes, the process of addiction can begin. Leventhal and Cleary (1980) have discovered that trying one cigarette does not generally lead to smoking, a comforting thought since many young people try smoking at least once. Curiously, however, by the fourth cigarette the addictive process is much stronger; a person who gets to the fourth cigarette is highly likely to become a smoker. Research has shown that smokers tend to be from two camps of teenagers; the most and least popular and successful (Mosbach and Leventhal, 1988). People with low self-esteem, or high self-esteem, people who are well-liked by peers or those who are not, and people scoring highly on class tests and people getting the lowest scores are the most likely to be smokers. Those falling in the middle of these extremes are less likely to smoke. This runs counter to the suggestion by Eysenck (1973) that extroverts are more likely to be smokers, since there is no reason to suppose that both groups of teenagers will be extroverted. Personality may be involved in smoking behaviour, however. There is some evidence that smoking can be a form of rebellion amongst teenagers who are inclined towards it (Jessor and Jessor, 1977). However, this does not explain the fact that smoking parents are more likely to have smoking children; it is difficult to use smoking as a rebellious activity when it is also a parental activity.

Smoking is a habit that is much more prevalent in working-class than middle-class people (GHS, 1999). On its own, the social-class distribution does not explain smoking behaviour. It is a useful way, however, to demonstrate how various factors can be interlinked. Working-class people tend to have working-class children, and middle-class people middle-class children. As a result, it is not possible to know whether certain people inherit 'addictive personalities' from their parents or whether there is something about social-class cultures which affects smoking behaviour in a more vicarious fashion. However, it is equally likely that the stresses felt by working-class people are dealt with by them by smoking. Although middle-class people experience stress too, the way that they choose to deal with it might be different from the coping mechanisms employed by working-class people. Indeed, since one group is financially better off than the other the ways in which they 'let off steam' may well reflect their disposable incomes. Therefore, whilst there is a strong social class effect on smoking behaviour, the reasons behind it are far from clear.

Smoking behaviour can sometimes be seen as an adaptive strategy, intended to reduce psychological stresses and thus as a health-giving behaviour, although a rather unusual one. Some people smoke to prevent stress, and to help them cope. A perfect example of this view is shown by the work of Graham (1998) who interviewed young women smokers with children whose main source of income was benefit. They often argued that they 'needed' a cigarette to calm down when children are crying, or when tempers are raised in the family. By smoking they may intentionally avoid, it is claimed, physical or psychological abuse of their children.

Work on the reasons why people smoke has uncovered some obvious answers and some less obvious. Some people simply claim that they like the taste of tobacco smoke, or the smell, or some other sensual property of the process of smoking (Leventhal and Avis, 1976). Leventhal and Avis also noted that smokers' self-reports of smoking behaviour centre around habit, addiction, or the properties of a cigarette to make a person feel more alert and attentive or to reduce anxiety and produce a sense of calm. Smokers often feel the need to smoke with a drink of alcohol or after a meal (Pomerleau and Pomerleau, 1989), something difficult to explain easily but worrying since if eating and smoking are somehow paired up there is a distinct encouragement to smoke every time a person eats. Since a smoker must eat, a smoker must therefore smoke.

Conditioning and smoking

The pairing up of smoking episodes with other events leads us now to briefly consider one of the views of why smoking is so difficult to stop doing. That is, the effects of stimulus–response association, or conditioning. There was a time not so long ago when psychology was dominated by the **behaviourist** or **associationist** approaches; both concentrated on the fact that human beings are animals and that we learn a great deal of what we learn, if not all, by means of nerve cells or groups of them learning to react in certain ways to things that happen to us. Essentially, we learn things by pairing a stimulus with a response, and usually a reward comes in somewhere. So, there was a time when you did not know what an apple was. You saw an apple, and your caregiver said the word 'apple'. Perhaps on a number of occasions this occurred, until you began to realise that there was a relationship between the word 'apple' and the object. You can start to use the word yourself at this stage. The stimulus is the apple (or the thought of an apple), and the response is the word 'apple'. The reward might be intrinsic satisfaction at having learned how to express something, or it might be a hug or a smile from your caregiver, or even an apple to eat. Either way, you have learned the pairing of the word and the object, and once learned these types of pairings are often unshakeable; that is why you still know the word 'apple' after many years. Common stimulus–response pairings in everyday life could include:

- hunger = eat food
- sound of breaking glass = look out!
- red traffic light = stop!
- leave the house = close the front door
- nearing house = reach for keys

People may smoke because they learn to pair up the act of having a cigarette with its effects, or with some other act or event. As mentioned earlier, smoking can increase alertness. If a person desires being alert, and a cigarette provides it, there is a stimulus–response association immediately set up. If a person associates smoking with being with friends and having fun, not only might they smoke when amongst friends, but also when alone and/or not having fun, in order to generate a feeling of bonhomie.

Giving up smoking

When psychologists deal with smoking by helping people to give up the habit, they sometimes do so by using conditioning. **Aversion therapy** is a form of this. In aversion therapy, an attempt is made to deter someone from smoking by getting them to concentrate on the negative aspects of it. Aversion therapy can come in weak or strong forms. A weak form would be allowing someone to smoke but expecting them to focus on unpleasant aspects of smoking, such as the burning smoke and its taste, whilst they do so. A stronger form would be forcing the smoker to smoke more than usual until they feel ill from it, known as **rapid smoking**. Repeated episodes of this 'oversmoking' can deter the individual from smoking permanently. Such drastic methods are rarely used any more since they are theoretically quite dangerous.

Conditioning is not the only way we have of helping people stop smoking, although there is often some element of conditioning, whether covert or overt, in many of the techniques which are used. The most basic form of anti-smoking technique is the health promotion campaign, aimed at groups rather than individuals. By warning people about the dangers of smoking, it is hoped that people will turn away from it. Indeed, there is evidence that such campaigns do work. Egger *et al* (1983) report the success of a three-year Australian media campaign in coastal New South Wales. The campaign had a threefold purpose; to stop people smoking, to get them to cut down on fat in their diets, and to get them to take regular exercise. The media campaign was extensive, involving radio and television advertisements, newspaper articles, T-shirts, stickers, and self-help kits. Two towns were enrolled, and one other served as a control town and ran no such campaign. In one town the media programme ran alone, and in the other the media programme ran with a community-based intervention scheme. In the joint programme, the best success was reported for young men (aged 18–25), for whom there was a decrease in smoking rates of 15.7%. The worst was for older women in the (over 65) for whom the figure was 6.1%. However, in the control town there was a decrease of as much as 5.1% over the course of the study, for women aged 18–25 and men aged 36–55. Therefore, we must essentially subtract the appropriate control decreases from the decreases observed from the towns enrolled in the media campaign. Doing this yields true declines in smoking rates of no more than 12.7% for men aged 18–25 and 4% for women over 65. Of course, a reduction of around an eighth in smoking rates in young men could have considerable benefits in terms of saving lives and resources in later years. What is clear from the Australian study is that no campaign at all is worse than a media programme, and that a community programme alongside a media campaign serves the purpose best of all. Of course, a shrewd reader may have spotted that the study lacks a useful comparison group. There was no town enrolled in the study who received a community programme but no media campaign. As a result, there is no way of knowing if the media-and-community group owed its success to the community intervention rather than the media campaign.

In addition, pressure can be put on smokers at the highest level by governments taxing tobacco products at a high rate, thus increasing their cost to the consumer. Whilst this might not prove to be a particularly strong deterrent for adults with incomes to cope with it, it might put off younger people, such as school children. Anti-smoking campaigns often try to frighten people away from smoking by associating smoking with its dangers. Taxing tobacco products makes smoking more of an unpleasant activity because it hacks away at a person's disposable income. These are examples of the most subtle forms of conditioning approaches; indeed, not all psychologists would agree that they are forms of conditioning in the most strict sense.

Today, most individual smoking-cessation programmes involve some combination of the different techniques. Generally, these combinatorial programmes work better than single techniques, and are more likely to last. One of the first steps in getting someone to give up smoking may involve a substitute way of introducing nicotine into the blood, without having to smoke tobacco. Nicotine patches and gum are a controlled way of doing this which have attracted much attention in recent years. There is substantial evidence that they can make a difference. An impressive meta-analysis of 17 placebo-controlled studies into nicotine patches was conducted by Fiore *et al* (1994). On average, 9 per cent of people wearing a placebo patch (containing no nicotine) gave up smoking, whereas 22 per cent of those with the genuine nicotine patch did. No-one knew which type of patch they were wearing.

Gourlay *et al* (1994) carried out a study to determine which factors were most important in the outcome of using nicotine patches to help people to stop smoking. They surveyed 1481 people who smoked at least 15 cigarettes per day. Over the six months of the data collection period, 316 of the participants stopped smoking. The most successful participants (in terms of quit-rates) were men, people over 40, those married or living with a partner, those having high motivation to succeed, and people who expressed concern over gaining weight after giving up. People who smoked marijuana were less likely to succeed in giving up (hardly surprising since the drug is often mixed with tobacco, and some people continued to use marijuana when enrolled in the smoking-cessation study). The most unusual finding is that people concerned about gaining weight were *more* likely, rather than less, to successfully quit. Weight-gain concerns are normally expected to deter people from stopping smoking. Perhaps, at least in the people in this study, concerns about gaining weight actually betray somatic knowledge, which could be implicated in successful health behaviour. If a person understands how their body works they might be more able to support it when required.

Allowing people access to nicotine via patches will certainly assist in the physical aspects of nicotine addiction, but will not serve to deal with the more psychosocial aspects, such as the environmental cues to smoke like stress and drinking coffee, pressure from smoking friends and so on. These require other approaches. A combination of techniques, such as nicotine patches, some self-help strategy, and some other intervention by a therapist or doctor is the most likely to work (Lando, 1977).

One particularly interesting factor in smoking behaviour relates to body-image. There is evidence that some young women smoke because they seek to have slim bodies and believe that smoking will enable them to achieve and maintain this (Ogden and Fox, 1994). Here, the smoking behaviour is clearly a means to an end rather than an end in itself. This shows that the appetites can often blend together in ways which psychologists can have mixed success in predicting. In a case like smoking to lose weight, nicotine patches are unlikely to have any impact on behaviour.

However, there is one more thing to consider. Psychologists do not need to be involved in helping *all* people to stop smoking; only some individuals require assistance. A lot of people can stop by themselves, using their own willpower, although it may take several attempts. Schachter (1982) asked smokers about their habit and found that over half of them had given up smoking entirely on their own, and since then had not touched cigarettes for years. This included very heavy smokers.

ALCOHOL

Alcohol is another legal drug which causes both health and social problems. Excessive consumption can lead to liver disease, heart disease, mental degeneration and cancers of the digestive tract. Alcohol is implicated in many violent acts against the person, and is, with chronic use, associated with reduced sexual appetite. It is said to be involved in 60% of suicide attempts, 30% of divorces and 20% of admissions to psychiatric hospital (Bennett, 2000).

It does not require much experience of the world to know that alcohol affects behaviour, and is a psychoactive substance. It depresses the action of the nervous system. People under the influence of alcohol speak more slowly and less well, they are less able to walk or perform co-ordinated hand movements, and their reaction times are considerably slower. Alcohol lowers inhibitions, so that people who are drunk may do and say things which they would not normally. They are more likely to embarrass themselves. People may take more risks when drunk, and are much more likely to injure themselves. That large quantities of alcohol are bad for the body is obvious the next day when people often report a 'hangover'; headaches, nausea, even tremors. This occurs because the body has, effectively, been poisoned. So why do some people regularly do this to themselves?

Like smoking, alcohol is something which often appeals to younger people, and so studies show that people often have their first experiences with alcohol as teenagers, and, often, before they are legally allowed to buy and drink it. In this sense, alcohol use reflects trends in smoking behaviour. In Britain, in an effort to prevent alcohol being made to look appealing to children, the law forbids advertising for alcohol products to show people who *look* under the age of 18, even if they are older.

Drinking to excess is something which is found all over the world, certain countries excepted, and there are regional trends in alcohol consumption and abuse. In Europe, French people drink a great deal of alcohol. As a result, deaths from cirrhosis of the liver are very common in France (Schmidt, 1977). Therefore, health problems related to alcohol will vary from country to country. When reading what follows, remember that the vast majority of research into problem drinking has been conducted in the Western world, principally in North America, Britain, and parts of Europe. What motivates a drinker in Scotland does not necessarily motivate one in Chile. As Napoleon (1999) explains, alcoholism amongst the Yup'ik Eskimos of Alaska may be a disease stemming from spiritual malaise due to historical, sociopolitical disenfranchisement of their people. It is unlikely that a health psychologist in Britain would or could make such a claim about English problem drinkers. In the extensively researched populations, alcoholism develops partly as a response to forms of stress, known as the **tension-reduction hypothesis** (Cappell and Greeley, 1987). People report needing a drink to relax, or to make them more sociable. Some people like the fact that alcohol lowers inhibitions, allowing them to 'let their hair down' and join in the fun. Alcohol does tend to work, and so further states of tension are treated with more alcohol.

Typically, problem drinking comes in two main forms: binge drinking and chronic alcoholism. The binge drinker may not be physically addicted to alcohol, but will regularly drink large amounts of alcohol during a night out. The chronic alcoholic is addicted to alcohol and may spend none of their waking life truly sober. Most of what follows in this section of the chapter refers to alcoholism: binge drinking has been much less extensively researched.

Intervening in alcohol abuse

As is the case with smoking, there are a number of ways in which alcohol abuse can be tackled, ranging from national strategies such as taxation and health promotion campaigns, to individual treatment programmes. The individual treatment programmes closely match those used with smokers.

Before an alcoholic can be treated, it is often necessary to engage in *detoxification* first. This is often referred to as 'drying out'. The individual is basically denied all access to alcohol for a period of time, until all traces of alcohol are out of the body and the symptoms of alcohol withdrawal (like tremors, hallucinations, nausea) have dissipated. Only then is the process of overcoming the psychological dependence likely to be productive.

Various conditioning techniques have been successful with some people. These may involve taking a substance which causes the person to vomit if they then drink alcohol, such as 'emetine' (technically known as an antidypsotropic medication). A typical alcohol aversion therapy would involve having regular alcoholic drinks after taking emetine by injection, and then the person would be sick after each drink. The aim is, of course, to make the person associate alcoholic drinks with bouts of vomiting, thus making them ill-disposed to further alcohol. Wiens and Menustik (1983) reported that over half of their patients stayed away from alcohol in the two years after the therapy. Another, more modern and less extreme, version of emetic therapy involves giving people a drug like emetine and simply explaining to them what is likely to happen if they drink alcohol. The aim here is to prevent any alcohol being consumed. This is not the same as normal aversion therapy, however, since the aim is not to associate alcohol with something bad by direct pairing up, but simply to scare the individual away from alcohol based on a 'stay away from it or else' view.

One rather famous and different way of dealing with alcoholism is that taken by Alcoholics Anonymous (AA). Here, people meet to deal with their drinking behaviour by sharing experiences and admitting to each other that they have made mistakes by becoming addicted to alcohol. The AA method seems to rely strongly on a social support mechanism, something which psychologists know can heavily influence health behaviour. New members talk to older members about their experiences, and tips about staying sober and free from alcohol are shared. Unlike many programmes established by psychologists and other health professionals, the AA do not believe in moderation as a key to controlling alcoholism; they argue that total abstinence is the only reliable way to stop people being alcoholics. Their rather 'confessional' approach seems to work for some people, although studies directly comparing this method with others are few and far between.

Since alcohol forms a very valuable coping mechanism for many people, programmes designed to wean people off alcohol must help the individual to find other means of coping, otherwise they are likely to fail. The approaches based on this ethos try to replace alcohol with a new set of coping skills. These include the social skills necessary to refuse alcohol when it is offered, and to avoid situations which tempt the individual or bring about cravings for alcohol. The whole programme is often framed with some kind of 'punishment' should it fail; this is known as **contingency contracting** (a contract based upon a contingency, i.e. a particular outcome). Here the therapist and patient enter into a contract with each other. There is a financial or other loss associated with failing to meet the demands of the programme. Therefore, there is a practical incentive for the person to keep in line with expectations. For those people who object to 'punishment' in these situations, one can just as easily imagine a *reward* for sticking to the programme, such as being given one's money back at the end. As is the case with giving up smoking, these combinatorial therapies are more likely to work than any single technique used in isolation. The success of behavioural approaches which include skills training is good, as demonstrated by Longabaugh and Morgenstern (1999) in a review of the evidence. They conclude that although the approach is not better than others when used in isolation, it is beneficial when used in conjunction with other therapies, such as treatment using general social skills training, self-help group activities and chemical therapies.

ILLEGAL DRUG USE

The use of illegal drugs such as marijuana, cocaine, heroin, amphetamine, and LSD is something which is culturally bound. The popularity of using illegal drugs waxes and wanes over time. In Britain, the first major influx of drug culture into the country was in the 1960s. Before that, Britain did not have a significant drug 'problem', except some considerable time ago when taking opium, related to heroin, was a common habit amongst certain sectors of society. Drugs vary massively in their effects. LSD and marijuana are used to generate hallucinatory states, cocaine is a stimulant to the nervous system, and certain abused drugs actually depress the nervous system (tranquilizers, for example). 'Ecstasy' (MDMA) is used to generate a feeling of euphoria and a sense of friendship and sharing with others. Deaths related to the use of this drug have been reported in the press worldwide. There is a wealth of evidence to show that use of illegal drugs can have significant negative effects on health. Whilst not every user of such drugs reports ill health as a result, it is by no means uncommon.

The writer William Burroughs (1956) spent some of his early life abusing a multitude of drugs, and wrote about his experiences in both fiction and non-fiction, including a piece published in the *British Journal of Addiction*. This represented an important turning-point in the move towards a psychosocial model of illness where the client is valued and their expertise given credence by health professionals. It was from this point that the lesson was learned that in order to help others we must listen to what they know about their problems, rather than simply apply our 'cures' to them. The patient or client can be seen as an expert on their own behaviour, at least in some senses.

It is true to say that the market for illegal drugs is largely centred on younger people. Generally, the same people are drawn to illegal drugs as to legal ones such as tobacco and alcohol. Heroin addiction is one of the best studied phenomena in this area of human behaviour. One of the things which surprises people the most is that heroin, which is often portrayed as the most dangerous and extreme of illegal drugs, does not have very high levels of physical dependency. Most of the addiction is, in fact, psychological. When people are trying to give up heroin use they go through a period of 'cold turkey' when the body is dealing with the withdrawal from the drug. The symptoms are very similar to an influenza-type illness. The psychological addiction to heroin is much more difficult to deal with. In fact, as William Burroughs (1977) pointed out, stopping using the drug is not difficult to cope with compared with the fact that once someone is through cold turkey they are often left feeling like they have nothing else. Because heroin addicts often effectively live for heroin, life being a succession of 'fixes', once the heroin is taken out of the life there can be a feeling like there is nothing left to live for. Replacing the heroin with a purpose is the hard task of drug rehabilitation workers.

Methadone

One of the means used for weaning people off heroin is the substitute drug **methadone**. This is used for a number of reasons, including the fact that it works similarly to heroin but can be produced under controlled circumstances. This reduces the dangers to the liver and heart that heroin poses, and which are partly due to potential impurities in it when purchased from illegal sources. It does not tend to produce a 'high', unlike heroin, and can actually prevent highs being experienced from heroin use, should a methadone user revert to the original drug. Ironically, methadone itself is an addictive drug, and some people become physically dependent on it just as they were on heroin.

Generally speaking, methadone treatment programmes do not work in isolation. Since heroin is psychologically addictive, psychological support is necessary. A combination of therapy and methadone prescription is most likely to achieve the aim of weaning a person off heroin. Since other drugs can interfere with the process, most drug treatment programmes will involve tests for other substances. There is no point in trying to get a person to give up heroin if they are also using other drugs such as cocaine. What may happen is a complicated interaction between the various drugs being used which leads to a suppression of the success of the programme.

Solvent abuse

Finally, it needs to be pointed out that the abuse of substances can extend beyond the substances normally classified as drugs. There has been a problem of solvent abuse in many parts of the world for a number of years. Teenagers, principally, can become 'high' from inhaling the fumes from certain glues and from the propellants in aerosols. The research into this is very scant. As such, the area of substance abuse represents a valuable field for future work.

SEXUAL HEALTH

This is essentially a number of related issues, stemming from the fact that sexual activity has, primarily, two purposes, which are pleasure and repro-duction. Recreational sex, as it is known, comes with a risk of reproduction. Depending upon the politics and the religious affiliations of various nations, it may or may not be an issue for health psychologists to consider contraception as a sexual health issue. In the UK, most of Europe, and the US, it is an issue, and since most health psychologists work in these areas of the globe it will be discussed here. The second big issue is that of sexual acts and practices which may be healthy or unhealthy for the individual. Sexual activity can be important to the individual in maintaining mental and physical health. Like any exercise, in moderation the body welcomes it. Mental well-being can be enhanced by sexual activity because it is often about feeling wanted and accepted by others. However, it can also be detrimental to the mind and body. Sexually transmitted disease (STD) can and does kill people, and injures many more (including making them sterile), and unwanted sexual experiences (either unwanted at the time such as rape or abuse, or on reflection later giving feelings of regret or shame) can cause significant strain on the individual. Why people do what they do has been the main interest of health psychologists, sociologists being more fascinated by the meaning of sexual activity for individuals and for society as a whole.

Contraception

Of course, the issues of contraception and of sexually transmitted disease are related, since some methods of contraception (principally the condom) also protect the individual against STD. Doctors and other health professionals, therefore, are often keen to promote the use of condoms because they have this double effect.

Health psychologists have been involved in the process of modelling the reasons why some people are happy to use contraception and others are not. Naturally, the most obvious answer to this question is that some people have moral or religious objections to it, and some do not. The Roman Catholic Church, presently, condones only the withdrawal (withdrawal of the penis from the vagina prior to ejaculation) or rhythm methods (avoiding sex during periods of heightened female fertility) of contraception. Therefore, for many adherents to this faith, contraception using condoms and pills represents an interference with the will of God that pregnancies should occur.

Contraception, including methods such as withdrawal, can be seen in terms of the issue of control. Ultimately, for people who wish to protect their bodies against disease and do not wish to reproduce, contraception is an issue of control and self-efficacy. It involves the people involved defeating the natural urge to engage in sex in the most convenient and quick way, that is unprotected. Of course, sex without any form of protection or contraception is exactly how it has been developed over the millions of years of evolution. As with other appetites, we are attempting to fight evolution when we use condoms, pills, sponges and diaphragms. It is a difficult contest. The control can lie with both partners or with one of them. However, sexual activity is a social activity that both partners must take responsibility for. Condoms are worn by males, and the contraceptive pill ingested by females, but this does not mean that women are not able to control condom-related sex (by saying 'yes' or 'no', as a minimum), nor are men unable to influence the taking or not taking of contraceptive pills (at the very least in terms of providing reminders so that the woman does not forget to take them).

Lowe and Radius (1982) suggested an early health-belief model (HBM) to explain use of contraception in young adults. The usual HBM factors were proposed, such as costs and benefits of using contraception, and perceived susceptibility to threat or risk. Therefore, with respect to condom use, benefits might include (depending on the level of knowledge the potential user possesses) protection against STD, and prevention of unwanted pregnancy. Costs could centre around issues such as reduced sensitivity and lack of spontaneity of sexual activity. Indeed, Fisher (1984) found exactly this: young males were often opposed to condoms for these reasons, and this negative attitude towards them was associated with avoidance of their use. In addition, these authors put forward a range of other relevant factors concerned with the context in which sex takes place such as the sexual relationship and sexual expectations set by peers and wider society. They suggested that sexual knowledge, knowledge about contraception, attitudes to contraception and previous experience were important in establishing use of contraception, as was self-esteem and the nature of the relationship in which sex was taking place (when salient).

However, attitudes may not directly link with behaviour. Phoenix (1989) interviewed 79 pregnant women aged 16–19 about their history of contraceptive use, and found that although 28 of them thought that it was important not to become pregnant, 17 had failed to use any contraception. Some said that they did not believe that they were likely to conceive, others that contraception was unwieldy or was difficult to obtain. Another interesting factor was a lack of faith in condoms coupled with health concerns about the contraceptive pill. Therefore, one health concern was effectively weighed up against another, although most doctors would argue that the most trouble-some option was the one actually chosen.

One useful way to view contraceptive behaviour follows a developmental path. It is sensible to accept that women's needs and attitudes to contraception, and therefore contraceptive behaviour, are likely to change during the lifespan, and not just in the obvious way that contraception *per se* is not needed after the menopause when a woman ceases to be fertile. Lindemann (1977) suggested that contraceptive use can be characterised as a 'career', which develops during a person's sexual life. This is divided into three main stages, the natural stage, the peer prescription stage and the expert stage. In the natural stage, often in the teenage years (but dependent on time and culture), young women are barely beginning to see themselves as fully developed sexual beings. Sex, if it happens, tends not to be planned for, and is carried out as a spur-of-the-moment activity. As a consequence, contraception tends not to feature at this stage. In the peer prescription stage, advice on methods of avoiding pregnancy is sought from friends, rather than from health professionals. Lay experiences form the basis for contraceptive behaviour. The incidence of the less effective methods, such as withdrawal and the rhythm method, is high in this stage. At this point, sexual intercourse is becoming more a part of the person's normal life. Finally, the expert stage represents the point when a person makes informed choices and plans for a sexual life, getting advice from doctors rather than friends and aiming to use the most effective methods available. Whitely and Schofield (1986) meta-analysed 134 studies of the use of contraception in teenagers and found that there was some evidence for the existence of a career model, but only in females. Males did not show this developmental trend. Of course, the fact that we find that women tend to be a better population in which to demonstrate contraceptive behaviour can be no surprise, given that pregnancy is something which occurs *to* women and has, arguably, the greater impact *on* women.

Abortion

Again, some people are opposed to abortion on religious and/or moral grounds. For those who are not, other factors influence their attitudes and behaviour. Health psychologists have not usually concentrated on abortion in their endeavours to understand health-related behaviour. There are three reasons why women may choose to abort a foetus. The first, which is rare but occurs, is as a form of last-resort contraception. Secondly there are the cases where doctors' advice is to abort because of potential harm to the mother carrying the child to full-term, or in cases where it is deemed that the child is severely disabled (a controversial situation). Thirdly, abortions mainly occur because of unwanted pregnancies, where the woman feels that she is not ready or able, physically, financially or emotionally, to have a child.

In this case, known as **elective abortion**, decisions are often made after considerable thought and with some degree of anxiety and distress to the pregnant woman. Many women do undergo distress after the termination has taken place, but this can be ameliorated if the woman feels supported by her friends and family and if the decision is effectively shared, that is if others have the same opinion. Adler *et al* (1990) have shown that post-termination anxiety is greater when the decision has been a difficult one to make.

Sexually transmitted disease (STD)

Sexually transmitted diseases show changes in their prevalence across time in populations. However, it is rare for any single STD to disappear from a population, meaning that all sexual encounters carry a risk of contracting any STD. Sexually transmitted diseases include HIV/AIDS (dealt with separately below), and syphilis, herpes, and gonorrhoea. Most health psychology has focused on this issue in relation to condom use, since condoms can protect against many STDs. This, however, overlooks STD transmission between lesbian women, for instance, for whom condoms are simply not applicable. Part of the difficulty in researching attitudes to sexual disease is that the research is conducted in the 'cold light of day', whereas the sexual behaviour being researched isn't. As health psychologists we construct elaborate models to understand why people think the way that they do, and what influences their decisions to protect their sexual health or to take risks. Now, here is an important point. Any model relying upon 'thought' as a factor may fall short of explaining behaviour, since, as Abraham and Sheeran (1994) suggest, people are usually aroused when engaging in sexual acts, and so are less likely to think clearly about what they are doing. Sexual arousal is, quite simply, distracting.

One issue worth mentioning here is that of delay. The taboo of STD may pose a problem for health services, since people may notice symptoms but fail to see their doctor for some time, perhaps because of feelings of shame. Leenaars, Rombouts and Kok (1993) demonstrated that over a quarter of a sample of over 800 people who suspected that they had STD waited for four or more weeks before seeing their doctor. Whilst there is value in waiting because the human body is capable of mending itself, and unnecessary strain on health services can be avoided this way, delays of too long can actually impede the healing process. Where there is an intimate body part involved, the risk of delay is greater.

Acquired immune deficiency syndrome (AIDS)

AIDS has been deliberately separated here from STD, since AIDS is not always an STD. Drug users who inject, people who have received blood and blood products such as plasma, and foetuses can become infected with the HIV virus, sexual activity not being a part of this method of transmission. The human immunodeficiency virus (HIV) transmits itself largely through contact between blood, vaginal mucus, and semen in any combination. The presence of wounds in the mouth, on the genitals, and so on, can increase its likelihood of transmission, especially sexually. In many countries such as the UK, AIDS has not become the epidemic that some people were predicting decades ago, partly due to the success of campaigns to warn people of the dangers of unprotected sexual intercourse, and perhaps partly due to medical advances which have meant that HIV infection is much less likely to lead to AIDS than it was when the disease was new to doctors. However, in many countries in Africa in particular, HIV infection is widespread (with around 80% of the world's HIV-infected people living in Africa). A combination of poverty, poor nutrition, lack of education about sexual health, high rates of prostitution (linked, of course, to poverty) and lack of medical resources can be blamed for this. If people cannot afford condoms and have not been told how HIV infection occurs, it is not surprising that the rates of transmission are high. In places where prostitution is one of a very small number of ways in which women (and men, of course) can make money to clothe, feed and protect their families, the HIV virus is more likely to be able to spread. Recent research by Fine (2000) has identified, however, a group of women prostitutes in one African community who appear to be immune to HIV infection. Doctors are now looking at ways of replicating this immunity in order to develop some kind of inoculation.

Mays and Cochran (1988) point out that the perceived risk from HIV infection and AIDS is, to many people, just one more risk in a world full of them. Their study of Black and Hispanic American women showed that AIDS was not a particular fear for them over and above the other social, political, and financial threats such women often face as part of their daily lives. Therefore, in a rank-ordering of challenges and threats, AIDS is often seen as a relatively distant one. This kind of logic clearly explains the fact that people who are prostitutes out of financial necessity may be willing to engage in unprotected sex with their clients. Sex without condoms usually attracts a higher fee than sex using them. The reasoning behind this may be as follows: 'If I do this, I *might* get infected with HIV. Chances are that this one encounter will not infect me, but it's a possibility. But I *will* get money for this, and I need money. I can be *certain* of feeding my family for the next week. If I don't feed my children, they *will* get ill and they *will* be taken away from me'. The priority-setting behaviour is, therefore, understandable in the circumstances. Another situation where risk-taking may occur is when drugs are involved. When sex is offered in exchange for drugs, HIV infection is often a minor consideration (Booth *et al*, 1991).

One of the ways in which health promotion campaigns may work is by frightening people into engaging in health-protective behaviours. The protection–motivation theory, which we discuss elsewhere in this book, incorporates fear into it as a driving force in determining health behaviour. So-called 'scare tactics' are increasingly common, and are often used in campaigns against drink-driving, with real footage from accidents and real victims or perpetrators telling their stories. One such campaign was run in Australia in the 1980s, involving images of the mythical figure 'The Grim Reaper' to publicise AIDS and create anxiety such that people would protect themselves (Rigby *et al*, 1989). It did not work. Whilst the campaign did increase awareness and knowledge, it did not have an effect on behaviour. Scaring people, or *trying* to, can have the opposite effect. Examples of the type of thinking that a scare tactic might engender could include the following.

- **Fatalism:** Gosh! We're doomed, so there's no point being careful. If it's going to get me, it will get me.
- **Recalcitrance:** If they think they can stop me doing what I do by threats and trying to frighten me, they're wrong.
- **Denial:** It won't affect me. This message is intended for someone else, really. I'm not at risk.
- **Rebellion:** I like danger. I like to question what I'm told. This is just encouragement to me.

Denial is a particularly strong phenomenon at times. Temoshok *et al* (1987) asked people in various US cities if AIDS was a health concern for them specifically. People in New York were most concerned by AIDS, with 52% of people admitting that it was a health concern for them, and people in San Francisco were the least concerned in the cities studied, with a figure of 33% 'yes' responses. There are, proportionally, more people in San Francisco who are HIV-positive than anywhere else in America. Of course, this does not mean that denial is the only explanation. In a city familiar with AIDS, knowledge levels about it are likely to be high, and, if behaviour follows knowledge, people in San Francisco might have perceived themselves to be relatively safe from AIDS because they knew how to protect themselves from HIV as best as possible. This is a reasonable explanation since Temoshok *et al*'s study also compared attitudes across sexualities: gay, straight, and bisexual men were surveyed. AIDS was perceived as a bigger problem by the gay and bisexual men, who also had more knowledge about it and reported a greater perceived susceptibility to it. However, perceived risk was not accompanied by changes in sexual behaviour, perhaps again reinforcing the 'denial explanation' of these results.

Scare tactics are particularly unlikely to work in isolation. Telling someone to do something or else risk death may be a good way to get across the solemnity of a situation, but does not provide them with any tools for the job. Someone may accept the message that condoms should be worn to reduce the risk of HIV infection, but may not know how to fit them or, more commonly perhaps, may lack the social skills needed to raise the issue of condoms with a partner. The fear of AIDS can actually be supplanted by the fear of doing the wrong thing in an intimate situation or feeling silly by making a nervous attempt to discuss protection. In addition, everyone is not equally assertive. Therefore, skills training and education are important. In Britain, initial scare campaigns with sombre images were followed up by TV advertisements where scenarios involving heterosexual couples were played out, showing that it does not have to be embarrassing or off-putting to talk about and use condoms, or that it is often advisable to avoid penetrative sex if condoms are not available. Thus, the aim is that people are frightened about the prospect of AIDS but are also vicariously able to learn about how to deal with intimate situations involving safer sex.

Getting individuals to change their behaviour to reduce the risk of ending up HIV-positive tends to centre around four main strands. As Stein (1990) points out, these are using condoms, selecting partners more carefully, limiting numbers of partners, and limiting type of sexual activity. Of course, these may be easier to intend than to carry out. Again, appropriate education is necessary. A person from a point of view of relative ignorance may not understand enough about condoms to use them. In some countries, condoms are expensive, and beyond the budget of poorer sectors of society. Some people might not know how to select partners. For example, if they do not have a good knowledge of AIDS, they might not know that avoiding sexual intercourse with people who inject drugs is sensible. Similarly, limiting partners may not be an option for a person who is living in a peer group for whom 'promiscuity' is the norm. Finally, limiting type of sexual activity can be difficult. Not only does this require that a person knows which activities are in the safer sex category and which are not, but it also implies that people have choice in what they do. A person who is subjected to violence should they fail to acquiesce in their partner's sexual requirements may not have the freedom to limit sex to non-penetrative acts. Equally, some HIV-infection is likely to occur through unwitting partners who have trusted their lovers to be monogamous when in fact they are not. In addition, Marks *et al* (1991) demonstrated that 52% of men who were HIV-positive did not tell their sexual partners about this. Control, and informed choice, therefore, are not always the appropriate terms to use in describing sexual behaviour and intentions.

The puzzle of 'barebacking'

Since the advent of AIDS, a significant amount of work has been focused on sexual health in relation to it. One interesting development of late is the discovery of 'barebacking'; this is the phenomenon where some gay men are rejecting the use of condoms to protect them against AIDS and other diseases and are taking the risk of unprotected anal sex (Williams, 2001). Many doctors believe that this is a particularly risky behaviour, and is more likely to result in HIV infection than is unprotected vaginal intercourse. Again, this is interesting since it presents a key challenge to health psychologists. How can we explain why men from a community so familiar with the threat of certain diseases are engaging in behaviours which could shorten their lives by decades? This kind of risky behaviour is, however, by no means confined to gay men. Sobo (1993) found that some HIV-positive women did not use condoms with their regular partners but did, however, during more casual sexual encounters.

As mentioned earlier, denial is a factor which could explain some of this behaviour. Another answer might be that people believe that doctors will soon be able to 'cure' AIDS, or eradicate HIV. Thus, they take a risk in the belief that by the time it affects them there will be something that doctors can do which in turn means that there is never a real threat. Research by Kalichman *et al* (1998) suggests that this is a common cognition. Bakker *et al* (1997) looked at attitudes to condom use in gay and bisexual men and found that the motivations of younger men were not the same as those of older men. In younger men, knowing someone with AIDS was influential on intention to use condoms, but in older men it was not.

The factor of danger is implicated in a number of ways in gay men's sexual behaviour, as suggested by Flowers *et al* (1999). Some gay men 'cruise' for sex, by visiting areas of parks which are known within the gay community as places to pick up other gay men. Sometimes, public toilets may be used, a phenomenon known as 'cottaging'. The men interviewed in this study admitted that the danger associated with this behaviour was not only weighed up against the benefit of finding sexual partners, but was also, sometimes, part of the thrill. For some men, there was a danger associated with unprotected sex, but there were two other principle threats identified. These are the risk of being raped or beaten by other men, and the risk of being arrested by the police. The threat of arrest was identified by at least one participant as being enjoyable. Clearly, understanding sexual behaviour involves understanding the perception of risk, since for some people sexual pleasure can be enhanced by risk. Whilst it may seem unusual to some people that others are willing to put themselves in danger, it begins to make more sense if the danger is perceived as pleasurable.

THE ISSUE OF RELAPSE

With all of the problems dealt with here, there is a concern that people will relapse into old behaviours once the 'treatment' or intervention is over. Marlatt and Gordon (1985) point out that there is a difference between a lapse (smoking one cigarette or having a sip of whisky before giving a speech) and a relapse (smoking an entire pack of cigarettes or drinking until quite drunk). However, to many people one lapse can be the trigger for a relapse.

People who lose weight often tend to gain it again. Some smokers start smoking again. Alcoholics often return to alcohol later in life. Sex offenders have a rate of recidivism after receiving help. The rates of relapse vary from person to person, from treatment technique to treatment technique, and so on. However, relapse tells us something. It demonstrates that it is often very difficult to change established patterns of behaviour, and, perhaps, that people behave the way that they do for a reason. If a person eats too much because they feel unhappy about themselves and food generates a sense of comfort, then dealing with the eating behaviour will not necessarily mean that the inner insecurity is affected. The real problems may be much deeper than the presenting problems, and unless we can identify what they are we may always experience rates of relapse that are higher than we are willing to accept. A multidisciplinary approach to health issues, involving health psychologists, clinical psychologists, psychiatrists and other professionals, might be costly but could prove effective.

COMBINING APPETITES

One important point remains. We must not forget that, although we have addressed the appetitive behaviours separately for ease of study, many of these appetites pertain to every individual at once, in combination. Many people eat badly, smoke, drink too much, and engage in sexual behaviours which could prove injurious to them, all on a regular basis. Therefore, there are additive effects of these. The body, and the mind, is rarely suffering from only one of these things at once. Furthermore, some of these behaviours lead to the others, or at least predispose a person towards them. A person who smokes is more likely to drink alcohol, and vice versa, at least in non-Islamic cultures. Of alcoholics 90% are smokers, according to one study (Istvan and Matarazzo, 1984). Coffee drinkers are also more likely to smoke and drink alcohol. Personality is important; a 'rebellious' nature might mean that a person who is raised to believe that drink and sex and drugs are immoral will indulge in drinking, drug-taking, and so on. We know that people who drink alcohol to excess are likely to have very poor diets with much of their daily energy intake coming from the ethanol in their drink; ethanol can also reduce the body's catabolism of fat, hence promoting obesity (Suter *et al*, 1992). Alcohol and other drugs can reduce inhibitions, which means that a person who is under the influence of one or more of them is more likely to risk themselves by indulging in practices which might expose them to the HIV virus, or, more commonly, to any number of other sexual diseases such as syphilis or chlamydia. Regular use of marijuana may cause a person to develop a poor diet and gain weight, because one of the effects of the drug is to deplete blood-sugar. As a result, people who are using marijuana develop strong hunger for snack-foods such as chocolate bars. This phenomenon is known to users of the drug as 'the munchies'. Those users who give in to the munchies are at risk from gaining weight.

Therefore, appetites do not exist in isolation. Psychologists need to understand the combinatorial, multivariate effects of appetites. By focusing on one at a time, they risk missing the 'bigger picture'. Sometimes behaviour is like a jigsaw puzzle. Looking at one piece at a time can be the way to build up that bigger picture. However, at other times it is like a book. It is meaningless if we concentrate on each word separately; we need to remember the previous words, and use them to help us interpret the ones we read next.

CONCLUDING REMARKS: SELF-HARM

One way in which the combinations of appetitive behaviours can be understood is by reference to the key issue of self harm. Ingesting a range of drugs and eating too little or too much or badly may be seen as forms of injury to the self. Self-harm is a major issue for doctors, and clinical psychologists and psychiatrists are very familiar with its manifestations. Many people clearly have a drive towards injuring their bodies in one way or another, which range from mutilation using broken glass or knives, through to tattoos and body piercings. Some authors argue that all of these behaviours, along with damaging appetitive behaviours, are forms of the same things: a desire to harm oneself. In understanding health behaviours, we must consider this common problem and build it into our models of why people smoke, drink, or eat to excess or until they starve. It may explain the apparent contradiction that people continue to engage in harmful behaviours even when they know that they are harmful.

Study questions

1. Would you say that you were addicted to anything, however slightly? What efforts have you made in the past to change your eating, drinking or smoking habits? Were they successful? Whether 'yes' or 'no', ask yourself why.

2. To what extent is addiction out of some people's control?

FURTHER READING

Marlatt, G.A. and VandenBos, G.R. (eds) (1997): *Addictive Behaviours: Readings on Etiology, Prevention, and Treatment*. Washington, DC: American Psychological Association.

   Collected reprints from journal articles on addiction. A good range of topics and approaches.

Nauta, H., Hospers, H. and Jansen, A. (2001). One-year follow-up effects of two obesity treatments on psychological well-being and weight. *British Journal of Health Psychology*, 6, 271–84.

   A comparison of cognitive and behavioural treatments for obesity. Noteworthy for the finding that even people who gained weight over the year of treatment showed improvements in psychological well-being.

7   Communication and Behaviour

- Introduction
- Patient–patient communication
- Professional–patient communication
- Recall of information
- Censorship
- 'Challenging' patients
- Professional–professional communication
- Communicating with children
- Written communication
- Concluding remarks
- Study questions
- Further reading

INTRODUCTION

If a doctor were to give you a pill to take twice a day, after meals, would you be certain of what you had to do? Which meals? Does breakfast count? What if the container label said that you could not take the drugs with milk or other dairy produce? You might avoid taking a pill after a bowl of cereal or a cheese sandwich, but what about milk in tea or coffee? Would that count? The seemingly most simple instructions can give rise to confusion. Exactly how doctors communicate advice to patients is an area of strong interest to health psychologists. So much success in the treatment of patients can be attributed to the minutes spent in giving appropriate information to them, and so much failure can be blamed on poor communication.

If a doctor is kind to you, polite to you, and listens to you, what do you feel? Is it different from what you feel if they are rude to you, cruel to you, and ignore you? The answer, of course, is yes. Doctors are people, and seeing a doctor is really only an interaction between two people. There is a power differential, there is a knowledge differential, there is a mediating social context, but at heart what is going on is that two people are communicating with each other. All of the standard 'rules' of communication apply. Whether you are old, young, male, female, rich, poor, highly educated and so on can all affect the nature of the interaction between you and your doctor, whose characteristics will interact with yours.

It is not surprising, then, that health psychologists have focused quite a lot of attention on communication in medical and para-medical settings. Psychologists know only too well how much the success of a meeting between people can be attributed to who says what to whom, when, where, how, and for how long. Doctors and nurses often report problems in dealing with patients, talking to them and conveying information to them, and, conversely, patients often complain about the interactions they have had with health professionals.

Davis and Fallowfield (1994) suggest that the communication problems which occur often involve the health professional making mistakes such as:

- not introducing themselves
- not asking for additional information or clarification from the patient
- not allowing or encouraging patients to ask questions
- not asking about patients' feelings, instead concentrating on medical 'facts' of the case
- not providing adequate information of a type that the patient can utilise.

In a sense, these are the kinds of problems that we might have predicted, since they are often the problems which can hamper any communication conducted with limited resources. The profusion of books aimed at enhancing communication skills for health professionals in the last 20 years or so is testament to the growing sensitivity to this fundamental aspect of healthcare provision. Indeed, Duxbury (2000) points to the sudden growth in books for health professionals about communication, and freely uses the term 'therapeutic communication'. Built in to this phrase is the implication that good communication is a key part of, and sometimes most of, the treatment of a patient.

PATIENT–PATIENT COMMUNICATION

Very little research has been conducted into the exchange of medical information from lay person to lay person. However, people often lay great store by their friends' and family's advice on medical matters. There is a literature available on folk remedies, and this shows clearly that some dangerous ideas about the way that the body works and the way to cure illnesses are spread around from person to person and are believed in and acted upon by individuals. Stacey (1988) distinguishes between formal and informal healthcare. The former is that provided by pharmacists, doctors, and related health professionals, and the latter is that provided by friends and family. She asserts that the majority of health care around the world is informal.

Mention should be made also of the sociological concept of a **lay referral network**. This is essentially the knowledge and social network of friends and family who consult with each other about health and illness (Friedson, 1960). For many people, such a network might be their primary source of information and decision-making about health issues. There is evidence to suggest that this is particularly strong in older people, at least in some societies (Stoller, 1984). As a consequence, doctors should be aware of the force of such a source of information, and the benefits as well as the drawbacks of its existence. Whilst some people will receive bad advice, others may get better as a result of the lay information exchange and any consequent self-help, and will thus place less reliance on health services. Given that older people tend to be ill more often than younger people, services might be noticeably more strained if the networks did not exist.

PROFESSIONAL–PATIENT COMMUNICATION

The vast majority of work on communication has been focused on doctors, nurses and other professionals communicating with patients. Just about every conceivable angle of these interactions has been studied, from the positioning of furniture in the consulting room, to the wording of leaflets given to patients inside packs of pills. The latter, written communication, will be dealt with separately later in this chapter.

When information is transmitted from one person to another, there are a number of points at which errors can occur. Not only might the doctor explain the information badly, but the patient may misinterpret what is said, and may also misremember it later. A combination of all of these means that the intended message can be quite different from the one the patient recalls. The knowledge gap between doctors and patients has been explored in a number of studies. In many respects, doctors and patients live in different worlds and speak different languages. Doctors may think that patients know more than they actually do. Doctors and other health professionals may be insensitive to ambiguities in their advice. For instance, Mazzulo *et al* (1974) showed that a large majority of patients would take various drugs at the wrong times and in the wrong circumstances based upon their understanding of the printed advice provided. Thioridazine labels suggested to patients that the drug should be taken three times a day. It was clear that some people interpreted this as meaning a 24-hour day, whereas others based this upon an interpretation of the 'day' as opposed to 'night', thus opening up a much shorter time period for the drugs to be ingested in. When unambiguous labels were provided, the numbers of correct interpretations of the advice rose dramatically. Hadlow and Pitts (1991) gave relatively common terms used in describing health, the body and health states to health professionals and to patients. Not only did they find that only a third or so of patients properly understood them, but also that a third of doctors and nurses did not. Obviously, this spells danger for the communication of such things from doctor to patient. A doctor who is less than *au fait* providing information to a patient who is confused is a recipe for disaster. The evidence we have, however, suggests that a proportion of medical encounters must be affected by problems like this.

Studies often look at both the nature of the interaction between professional and client, and the time spent in interaction. In addition, the level of client satisfaction with the encounter is a common measurement, along with, in the more clearly psychological studies, some index of how well the information imparted has been understood and remembered. Here we concentrate on a selection of factors involved and the research conducted into them. In considering these, it is essential that we remember that any one of these in isolation is unlikely to be a key factor, and that a combination of these is what makes up a person. It is, after all, a person that the doctor communicates with.

Age

As we age, our abilities change. Many of them wane over time, but we tend to become better communicators, in the sense that our vocabularies expand. However, our memories tend to become significantly worse. Therefore, on the simplest level, doctors communicating with older patients are generally more successful if they can deliver a message which the patient can remember. A memorable message for a 20-year-old is not that different from a memorable message for a 70-year-old, except perhaps in degree. Therefore, if you aim to deliver a short, pithy message to a younger person, it might need to be shorter and more pithy for the older one.

There is a wealth of literature to substantiate the claim that task complexity and age interact, such that the more complex a task becomes the more disproportionately difficult it becomes for older people. This has also been shown in the health adherence literature. Kiernan and Isaacs (1981) studied the recall of dosage information for people over 65 and found that it became more and more unreliable as the number of drugs to be taken in a day increased. Furthermore, people are more likely to forget to take drugs when they are taking a collection of substances rather than one or two.

In most societies, age is related to forms of culture. People of different ages are essentially people of different cultural groups. (Naturally, this is *on average*. Not all people fit their age stereotypes by any means.) Therefore, when doctors and patients differ in age, they may also differ in values, attitudes, ways of viewing the world, interpretations of reality, knowledge about the body and how it works, morals and so on. For more information on communication in relation to age, look at the section on communicating with children further into this chapter.

Gender

It is seemingly obvious that the patient's gender, and that of the professional, are likely to interact in ways which may enhance or inhibit communication. Doctors are more likely to view women as hypochondriacal, and to take men's health issues more seriously than women's. For example when men and women present to doctors with colorectal cancer symptoms, men get a final, exact diagnosis earlier than women (Marshall and Funch, 1986). Such inequalities stem from gender-based attitudes, and those attitudes can shape the interaction between patients and doctors. Feminist writers often speak of the 'medicalisation' of women, and how the traditionally male-dominated medical profession has involved itself in the ordinary aspects of women's lives (menstruation and childbirth, for instance), and taken over control in such areas (Oakley, 1980). In particular, Oakley noted how doctors often tended to argue with pregnant women over the expected date of birth, as if the women could not have any expertise on this issue. When women asked about pain and discomfort, as they did in 12% of questions, they were dealt with by mainly dismissive remarks from the doctors. Such exchanges serve to make women less confident in their doctors.

Socio-economic status

How much money a person has, and their social standing, can also impact upon the healthcare they receive, including the communication with health professionals which can occur. To cite an example, Blair (1993) used a socio-linguistic framework to investigate the nature of communications between doctors and their working-class or middle-class patients. Working-class people are more likely to use terms associated with physicality when talking to their doctor, whereas middle-class people used terms related to mental health and the psyche. Therefore, the working-class patients would focus on aches, pains, constipation and so on, whereas middle-class people would refer more often to depression, anxiety, stress and the like. In terms of treatment, working-class people saw physical interventions as the best answer for their problems (drugs and surgery), but for middle-class people there was a greater interest in counselling, psychotherapy, and other, less formal non-physical interventions. There are a number of possible explanations for this. It might be that people from different socio-economic strata actually develop different symptoms and illnesses. A person whose work is mainly manual (a working-class person who is a gardener or a road-mender, for instance) may be more likely to injure their body than their middle-class counterpart, such as a lawyer or lecturer. But, there may be greater mental stresses placed upon the person who is middle-class than on the working-class individual. However, there could also be an effect of education. It might be that a working-class person, who almost by definition is less likely to have the educational history that a middle-class person does, is simply less aware that a doctor's role is to assist in all aspects of health, not just physical health. Equally, there may be a cultural taboo of mental illness in operation which affects working-class individuals much more than those from the middle-class. At the moment, this is merely supposition, since little research has been done which tests these hypotheses against each other.

Ethnicity

The consideration of ethnicity as a factor influencing doctor–patient communication is much wider than the simple issue of language. It is true that doctors may vary in their command of the language they are using, especially if they are not using their mother tongue, and the same applies to their patients. However, more subtle (but not necessarily less important) effects inhere in the cultural differences and attitudes that exist.

What is said in the consultation is no more important than what is not said. McAvoy and Raza (1988) studied Anglo-Asian women's attitudes to contraception, and found that although many doctors would not offer it to them because they assumed it did not fit with their culture, a high proportion of them had used contraception and were in favour of its use. Thus, doctors must cast off their own prejudices and stereotypes about Asian women and sensitively and appropriately offer them the full range of services available to all patients, letting the person decide for themselves if it is relevant for them. Remember, however, that we are not only dealing with non-Asian doctors potentially holding stereotypes about Asian women. Doctors from the same background as the women may also make assumptions about their lifestyle and beliefs.

Consultation time

A clear finding is that more time spent does not mean better information-transfer nor greater patient satisfaction (Korsch and Negrete, 1972). Satisfaction with duration of consultation is moderated by the patient's experience of the nature of the consultation. If patients have been given the opportunity to express themselves and ask questions, they tend to be satisfied with the length of the consultation, even if it is short. Of course, patient satisfaction is a highly sought after thing, and satisfied patients do tend to experience (or at least report) less pain and are easier to 'cure', as judged by less time spent in hospital.

Consulting style

Savage and Armstrong (1990) conducted a rare 'true experiment' into the style adopted by the doctor and its effects on the level of satisfaction with the consultation reported by the patient. Just prior to seeing a patient, doctors were randomly assigned to behave in one of two ways: in a sharing fashion, or in a directive fashion. Sharing styles involve the patient in the consultation, creating knowledge by asking them questions, whereas directive styles are more about imparting information of which the patient is a recipient. The authors found that, contrary to what one might imagine given the modern trend towards co-operation between patient and doctor in achieving health, directive styles created more patient satisfaction than sharing ones. This was a clear effect in patients who had a physical rather than a mental illness, and in patients who rarely saw their doctor. Thus, one can see that this suggests that when people want a 'no-nonsense' diagnosis and some direct treatment advice for a simple physical illness, the directive style is better. Some people do not want the doctor to *ask* them what is wrong with them, they want to be *told* what is wrong by the doctor. Additionally, because the people who attended rarely were best suited to a directive style, this implies that those people who attend regularly might need to feel that the doctor is sharing information with them, is listening to them, and is involving them in all stages of the case. The study demonstrates that a 'one-size-fits-all' approach to medicine simply does not work. Tailored care is more appropriate, and our attentions should be focused on identifying, quickly and easily, which patients are best suited to which approach.

There is evidence to suggest that health professionals use age-inappropriate language codes when talking to patients. This can be perceived by patients as a patronising, condescending style. The language of health professionals is often similar to that used by adults when talking to children. As Toynbee (1977) first remarked, doctors and nurses' talk is replete with 'baby-talk' terms such as 'slipping' and 'popping'. People are asked to 'pop' off their clothes and 'slip' into a hospital gown. They have 'bums' and 'tummys', and operations involve taking a 'peep' and making a 'snip'. People are asked to 'wee' rather than to urinate to produce a sample. Similarly, some readers will be familiar with the rather unusual grammar often adopted by health professionals, which can involve the omission of possessive pronouns with the effect of creating an artificial intimacy between patient and health professional: 'Remember to feed baby later . . .', 'How is Dad today?', and 'How are *we* this morning?' Some argue that this kind of linguistic style represents infanticisation, the reduction of an adult to the status of a child. Naturally, some patients are likely to resent this. Equally, patients may have some difficulties with heavily jargonistic language too. If doctors use too many technical terms, patients are confused, naturally. If health professionals can find a balance between simplistic and esoteric language, patients are most likely to benefit from the consultation.

RECALL OF INFORMATION

One of the best ways to measure success of communication is in how well the information imparted is remembered. Ley (1989) summarises the research into communication and recommends the following to maximise the amount of information remembered by patients when it is provided to them by doctors and nurses.

- People tend to remember the things which they are told first, rather than those things which are presented later in the conversation. This is known to psychologists as a primacy effect. Doctors can make use of this by putting forward the key points earlier in the consultation. Saving the best until last is unlikely to make the impression intended.
- People remember short, pithy 'sound-bites' rather than complicated sentences containing long or jargon words.
- Repeated information is better remembered, something that psychologists call rehearsal.
- Specific, rather than general, information is more likely to be remembered. Therefore, talking about the patient and their particular case will be better than making more vague comments about 'people' who have 'similar' health problems to the patient.
- If the information is presented in categories which are clearly demarcated, recall is enhanced. Therefore, the information-transfer can be broken down into sections on diagnosis, treatment, self-help, and prognosis. The information should be given in this order. For example, the doctor might say 'You have hypertension. I can give you some drugs to reduce your blood pressure. You can help things along by avoiding foods with a lot of salt in them, and by losing a bit of weight. If the drugs work, and you manage these things well, you should be back to normal blood pressure within six months or so, and it ought to stay there after that.'

CENSORSHIP

There is some evidence that doctors may censor bad news so that patients do not always receive the truth about things that are happening to them (Nichols, 1993). This may be done for two reasons; firstly, the doctor might be aiming to shield the patient from information which they feel might harm them. Indeed, under current English law a doctor may withhold any information from a patient which, in their opinion, would harm the patient, either physically or psychologically, should it be disclosed (Montgomery, 1997). However, another reason might be because the task of giving very bad news is an unpleasant one which, sometimes, a doctor might feel unable to tackle. Censoring bad news is generally a poor way to communicate. It is often done in subtle ways by implying that a patient has more hope than they really have, or by leaving out some of the more anxiety-provoking details of the course of an illness. Ultimately, the patient is often disappointed because things turn out worse than they were led to believe, and they might then turn to viewing the health professionals involved as untrustworthy, incompetent or negligent. Honesty is usually the better policy, it seems.

Multiple sclerosis (MS) is a progressive disease which involves degeneration of the myelin sheath surrounding nerve cells. It occurs more readily in people who live further away from the equator. As a result of MS, the person slowly loses a number of bodily functions. Visual disturbance is common, movement is affected, and the patient will normally become incontinent. MS tends to be a spasmodic disease, going through a cycle of relapse and remission, each phase lasting often unpredictable amounts of time. It is a disease which, although not immediately life-threatening, can eventually lead to death and can certainly disable the individual significantly. As such, it is a difficult, emotive diagnosis to communicate to a patient. Elian and Dean (1985) spoke to patients who had been diagnosed with MS, 167 in total. They found that 18% of them did not know anything about MS, 19% had guessed what their diagnosis was without being told by a doctor, and 24% had been told by a doctor who was not the same consultant who had made the diagnosis. Furthermore, 6% of people had found out about their MS by accident, perhaps by overhearing conversations or from a hospital cleaner. Only 27% of people were told about their MS directly by their consultant without having to ask. It is clear, then, that the ideal situation where the doctor making the diagnosis clearly tells the patient about the illness does not occur in a sizeable proportion of cases. The researchers also found that 83% of patients interviewed did want a direct and clear explanation from the consultant, even though just over a quarter of them actually received this.

'CHALLENGING' PATIENTS

We must not forget, however, that the success of an interaction can be heavily influenced by the personal characteristics of the client no matter how the doctor behaves, and that some people present serious challenges which the most skilled health professional may find difficult to deal with. It is important to accept that sometimes the best doctors are simply faced with patients who communicate badly, whatever approach is used. Whilst it is the responsibility of the health professional to endeavour to communicate well with a client, it is not their responsibility to *succeed* in all cases. Sometimes success may prove virtually impossible. Duxbury (2000) shows that some clients are aggressive, perhaps violent, and many are persistently uncommunicative. If doctors take all available steps to work well with patients, this is as much as can be asked of them.

However, Jeffery (1979) points out that some very negative attitudes towards patients can be displayed by health professionals, even when the patients themselves are not particularly aggressive or challenging. Cases which health professionals do not particularly want to have to deal with have been reported as having been described by doctors as 'rubbish'. These include people with health problems which the doctors or nurses consider trivial, drunken people, homeless people, and those people who have taken overdoses of drugs which indicate attention-seeking behaviour or self-harm rather than genuine attempted suicide. Naturally, such strong opinions on the part of the hospital staff cannot fail to affect the way that they deal with these patients, regardless of the patients' actual behaviour towards the hospital staff.

PROFESSIONAL–PROFESSIONAL COMMUNICATION

Most health psychology concerns itself with doctors giving information to patients, but as much confusion and error can arise from the exchange of information from health professional to health professional. Faber *et al* (1991) outline a case of patient death resulting from the confusion of Losec and Lasix on a prescription due to a misreading of a doctor's handwriting. Many drugs have similar names, and many are therefore confusable in speech or writing. This is despite the fact that drug companies aim to avoid confusions when naming drugs (Holm and Evans, 1996). There has been a substantial shift towards the use of computer-printed prescriptions throughout the developed world as a result of this kind of confusion, but doctors who are on-call, visiting patients at their homes, still have to rely on handwritten prescriptions.

COMMUNICATING WITH CHILDREN

The history of doctors' dealings with children is not unlike communication in the veterinary profession. Communicating with children is often substituted for communicating with parents, just as communicating with animals is synonymous with communicating with their owners. That this is not satisfactory is outlined by Eiser and Twamley (1999) who point out that whilst parents might be good at giving details of what happened to the child, they may be less accurate in describing their child's feelings about what happened. Of course, children are not animals, and are often able to express their feelings and thoughts, albeit in ways different from those employed by an adult. The challenge for paediatricians, and for all health professionals, is in understanding children and combining their answers with information provided by their guardians to achieve an accurate diagnosis.

Although children do have ideas and thoughts of their own, there is some evidence to show that their illness cognitions are affected by those of their parents. Children learn so much from their parents that it is hardly surprising that they pick up ideas about their own health status vicariously. Walker *et al* (1991) demonstrated that parents with a chronic health problem were more likely than those who do not to have children who see a doctor because they are experiencing abdominal pain. The pain is often unexplained, suggesting that the child might be imitating the parental behaviour.

Developmental stages

Quite simply, children do not think about health and illness in the same way that adults do (Bibace and Walsh, 1979). They have different conceptions of their bodies, and so need to have their needs addressed in their own ways. Bibace and Walsh have identified six stages that children may go through in their understanding of the relationship between health, the body's functioning, and individual behaviours.

- **Phenomenistic stage:** When infants initially develop a view of the causation of illness, it tends to be phenomenistic. This means that there is a focus for causation in one observed thing. The child may link this phenomenon with disease without there being any obvious association to an adult. Therefore, an infant might believe that toothache is caused by an armchair, perhaps because they were sitting in the chair when they first experienced toothache. Just as infants tend to generalise or be too specific in their use of language, so they might also do this with respect to their understanding of illness. They might believe that all armchairs cause toothache, or rather that it is only caused by the armchair in their home. Another common example of this mode of thinking would be the claim that God causes illness. In addition, illnesses tend to be defined by a single symptom, rather than a constellation of them. Therefore, a cold is a runny nose, heart disease is a red face, or diabetes is being fat. This mode of thinking tends to dominate the first few years of life.
- **Contagion stage:** From the ages of around three to seven years, there is a growing acceptance that disease and illness can be passed on from person to person, or from things to people. However, there is little more sophistication than this. The child may tend to believe that *all* illness is contagious, asserting that people with cancer can give you cancer if you stand near them. The definition of 'near enough' to be 'infected' can vary. Some children may believe that you have to be touched, others that standing near to the person would be enough. Oddities like a belief that speaking on the telephone could transmit disease can be observed in some children.
- **Contamination stage:** This is a development from the contagion stage. Here children have started to accept that illness is often associated with a range of

symptoms, and that our behaviour is implicated in how healthy or ill we are. Instead of believing that disease is somehow magically transferred from person to person, there is evidence of agentive reasoning. The children are implying that they know that disease is borne by an agent, such as the air, and that germs and viruses are involved. This stage of understanding is normally prevalent around seven years of age.

- **Internalization stage:** In this stage, a key characteristic of the child's thinking is that they have some responsibility for their health by behaving in certain ways and engaging in certain acts and avoiding others. There is a view that illness and disease are about the body, and things happening inside the body. The child is also beginning to understand the rather sophisticated notion that behaviour can be directly involved in ill health. At this stage, children may have begun to say things like 'smoking hurts your body' and 'people who shout a lot and get angry can get pains in their heart.' This level of thinking develops between the ages of seven and eleven, on average.
- **Physiological stage:** At this point, usually around eleven years of age, children, perhaps through increasing education, have a conception of the body being made up of organs which have specific functions, and they see disease and ill-health as being related to the dysfunction of organs and processes. They tend to be more likely to appreciate the fact that there are multiple causes of ill health.
- **Psychophysiological stage:** In this stage of thought, there is a proper grasp of the interplay between the physical and the mental in determining health status. In this stage, the child (who by now is probably somewhere between 12 and 14 years of age) realises that stress, for instance, is something which can lead to a variety of health problems, and that health problems can lead to stress.

As can be seen from the above, interpreting what children say about illness and their bodies should be undertaken using knowledge of the phases through which children pass on their way to 'mature' reasoning. What might seem as a perfectly sensible way to describe something to an adult may make no sense to a child. Since children who are ill essentially have the right to have procedures explained to them, doctors who can do so effectively are those who can speak to children on their level.

However, we must not forget that the stages outlined by Bibace and Walsh (1979) for children's understanding of health issues are not exclusively descriptive of childhood reasoning. It is not just paediatricians and the like who could benefit from a reading of research of this nature. All health professionals, including those who deal with adults, should be aware of the processes through which developing minds form conclusions. This is so important because a proportion of adults, principally those with learning disabilities, are operating at an intellectual level akin to children in these stages.

Collecting information from children

Collecting data or information from children can be achieved in a number of ways. Useful methods employed in the past have been drawing and play. By involving the children in acts which they normally engage in, the scene is set for an exchange which can be fruitful. Pridmore and Bendelow (1995) examined the beliefs about illness and death of children from Botswana, using a method involving both drawing and writing. They discovered that the children tended to blame supernatural beings for death, an explanation readily available in their culture.

Children and death

For children who are dying, communication is a particularly difficult issue for doctors. There are many debates over whether it is appropriate to tell a child that they are about to die, and how to do it. Some children will benefit from honesty, but others will have their remaining life affected by this knowledge. What Spinetta (1974) claimed was that terminally ill children were generally not told as much as adults in the same position, but, like adults, they were able to infer things from their physical state and the behaviour of others to make judgements about their health, even though adults around them tend to view them as naïve children. Keeping children in a state of ignorance can, some would argue, be seen as a contravention of their human rights.

Kane (1979) gives some useful information on children's concepts of death. Very young children tend to view death as a possible temporary state, and one which may include some consciousness or movement. She reports that the adult conception of death as an irreversible and all-inclusive phenomenon starts to become fixed at around six years of age, perhaps earlier than many adults would believe. However, it is only at around 11 or 12 years of age that some of the finer points associated with death become common knowledge to children, such as the nature of the physical processes involved and the emotional aftermath. The understanding of death can depend on experience. As Judd (2000) points out, children on hospital wards who have witnessed or at least been cognisant of the death of another child are much more likely to have an accurate picture of what death entails. If the child who has died did so because of an illness which the witnessing child also has, the effect is greater.

Interacting with children

The nature of the information gained from children, or their behaviour, may be a direct consequence of the behaviour of the adults they are engaged with.

Children may 'feed off' adult behaviour, especially adults they respect or are fearful of, such as parents and, of course, doctors. An excellent example of this comes of a study conducted in dentistry. Wurster *et al* (1979) categorised the behaviour of senior dental students into three types and that of their child patients into another three. By looking at videotapes of interchanges between the students and patients at very frequent intervals, judges decided whether the students were guiding, permissive or coercive. Similarly, they judged the children's behaviours as either co-operative, resistant, or unco-operative. They then looked at the associations between these different communication styles in student and patient. Firstly they considered what the children did after what the students did. They found that a guiding style tended to be followed by co-operation, but that coercive behaviour was nearly always followed by the child refusing to co-operate (defined as behaviour which interfered with the process of treatment). However, it is not this simple, since as you might have thought, behaviour is a two-way process. Therefore, it is difficult to say that the children's behaviour was a direct *consequence* of the dental students' behaviour; perhaps the students were responding to behaviour by the children. A further analysis looked at the behaviour of the students occurring *after* the behaviour of the children. Here it was found that co-operativeness in the children was followed by a guiding style from the student almost without exception, but that unco-operative behaviour was more likely to be followed by coercion (threats and so on) or permissiveness (giving in to the child being 'naughty') on the part of the dental student. This demonstrates, then, that the analysis chosen can determine the result, but that the 'truth' of the situation is probably somewhere between the two angles of approach chosen by the authors. The relationship between the dentist and the patient is a reciprocal one: it is very unlikely to be all about one person responding to the other all of the time, even if a lower-power individual, such as a child, is involved.

Stranger fear/stranger anxiety

A key issue in understanding the anxieties of children and how their concerns may prevent good communication and, therefore, good treatment is the notion of stranger fear. Just as Bibace and Walsh's (1979) cognitive–developmental approach to children's understanding of illness identifies stages through which children progress, there is a loosely developmental elaboration of stranger fear, describing stages through which infants move in their relationships with non-familiars. Put simply, very young babies tend not to have a concept of a stranger, but then by about seven months they are beginning to develop a feeling that there are people that they know and trust and that other people are, by default, not known and not to be trusted (Berk, 2000). Hence, children of around 1–2 years can be very hostile towards and afraid of others, especially adults. Stranger anxiety can be intense, and dissipates in children at different ages. Some children lose this quite early, around four years, whereas for others it can remain until around five or six years. Most of us will have met a child who hides behind its parents when strangers are around.

This phenomenon is as strong when the adult is a health professional as when they are not, and physical examinations by a doctor or nurse may prove particularly anxiety-provoking for the infant. In particular, it is not easy to explain to a small child that a person who is pulling their broken arm, or is prodding their wounded leg is 'trying to help them'. The evidence of their senses seems to suggest otherwise.

WRITTEN COMMUNICATION

Providing patients with written explanations of drug regimens or treatments or self-help techniques has been shown by a great many studies to enhance the success of communication, both in understanding and later recall.

Patient anxiety can be reduced by the appropriate use of written communications. Jackson and Lindsay (1995) made significant reductions in dental patients' anxiety prior to their consultation by giving them a leaflet which explained that the dentist would be willing to stop the procedure underway if they signalled to them that they did not wish it to continue, either because they were uncomfortable, worried, or in pain.

On the negative side, however, the good effects of written communication are not universal. Ley (1997) makes the assertion that up to a quarter of medical leaflets would be understood by as few as a third of the people that they are given to. Newton (1995) has shown that many leaflets made available to dental patients are not understood by them. We must bear in mind that health professionals are educated and literate, and may underestimate the reading skills of people less educated and less literate. In Britain, some of the most popular daily newspapers require low levels of literacy in their readers, akin to the reading ages of children, when readability formulae such as those of Flesch (1951) are applied to them. When the same formulae are applied to patient information literature, the discrepancy can be large.

With the increasing realisation that written communications do not always lead to greater understanding or satisfaction, alternative methods of information-provision are being experimented with by doctors, health educators and promotors, and, of course, health psychologists. Video is becoming a popular medium, for example. Tattersall *et al* (1994) looked at providing cancer patients with consultatory information either in the form of a letter or on audiotape. Whilst both formats produced equivalent levels of recall of the information contained within them, patients preferred the audiotape, thus creating greater satisfaction. Hogbin and Fallowfield (1989) gave breast cancer patients recordings of consultations where details of the 'bad news' of a positive cancer diagnosis was being outlined. Patients reported that the tapes helped them to understand their illness, increased their confidence, and helped them tell their friends and family what was happening to them. Therefore, when the information being presented is very sensitive and is likely to have serious consequences for the patient, some form of back-up that the patient can listen to repeatedly is likely to be extremely useful. Telling a person that they have cancer is usually extremely distressing for them. It is almost certain that any information imparted during the spoken consultation *after* the diagnosis has been given is likely to be listened to much less carefully than is necessary or desirable, simply because a distressed person cannot concentrate well. (If you are reading this book with something important on your mind at the moment, think about how easily you are distracted away from the text by your worries.) Audiotapes may be seen as preferable to written communications because they present information with a more 'human' touch.

CONCLUDING REMARKS

The reader would be forgiven for assuming that, given the vast amount of research which has been conducted into the realm of communication, there is nothing left to research. However, much remains to be done. Most research in communication, like most research in general, has been conducted with white British or American participants. The world contains many more people than this. Since communication is sensitive to culture, culture-specific studies are required. One individual difference which can influence the success of communication is dyslexia. Large numbers of people are dyslexic, and as yet no published material exists on whether dyslexia can affect communication with doctors. Are dyslexic people more likely to confuse one pill for another, or take wrong numbers of pills? Might they forget what the doctors have told them, since memory problems are associated with dyslexia? There are hundreds of studies on this alone waiting to be conducted.

Study questions

1. Would you be happy with a computer doctor instead of a real one? Whatever your answer, list your reasons.

2. Not all aggressive people choose to be so. Sometimes, their physical or mental illness creates their aggression. What are their rights to treatment, in your opinion?

FURTHER READING

Ley, P. (1988): *Communicating with Patients*. London: Croom Helm.
A 'classic' book on communication by the world's foremost researcher in the field.
Strydom, A., Forster, M., Wilkie, B.M., Edwards, C. and Hall, I-S. (2001): Patient information leaflets for people with learning disabilities who take psychiatric medication. *British Journal of Learning Disabilities*, 29, 72–6.
A paper looking at the nature of written communication and those people who have additional requirements which are not currently met.

8 Psychometrics and the Measurement of Health and Illness

- Introduction
- Internal reliability (internal consistency)
- Measurement scales
- Scales and sub-scales
- Validity
- Reliability
- Does 'off the shelf' mean good?
- Using tests
- Concluding remarks
- Study questions
- Further reading

INTRODUCTION

Psychologists are interested in what people do, and why people do what they do. The first of these is behaviour, and the second we might call motivation or impctus. Ideally, we need to be able to measure both of these. Measuring behaviour is relatively easy, because we can, mostly, use conventional tools. If we want to measure smoking behaviour, we can ask people to keep a diary of how often they smoke and where and when. If we want to know if a person is stressed, we can measure their heart-rate, blood pressure or skin conductivity (galvanic skin response or GSR). Of course, knowing how much or when a person smokes or how stressed someone is when they are at work does not tell us *why* they smoke, or what is happening at work to make them stressed (or, if you like, why they 'allow' events to stress them).

For this information, we turn to tests and surveys. In psychology, tests vary from the plain and simple to the long-winded and complicated. A 'test' of reaction time usually involves nothing more than pressing a button as soon as a sound is heard or a symbol appears on a screen. Sometimes a *series* of tests is necessary to get a picture of a person and their abilities or behaviours; a collection of tests, usually designed around one theme or purpose, is called a *battery*. There are a number of specialist terms which are used to describe tests. Most health psychology involves using questionnaires. For the purposes of this chapter, the terms questionnaire, test and instrument are used interchangeably. Tests which are researched and published, usually with extensive norms available, are sometimes called 'off the shelf' tests. This contrasts with home-made tests and questionnaires which must be produced when you are researching something totally new. 'Off the shelf' tests begin life as home-made tests.

In health psychology, a lot of test instruments involve a set of questions which have been designed to discover something about a person and their behaviours. People might be forgiven, when looking at a test, for thinking that it is easy to create. After all, there is a lot of common sense behind the questions. If you want to know how much value people place on having a healthy heart, asking them if they exercise or avoid fatty foods is sensible. But, just because these tests make good sense does not mean that common sense is all that is used to devise them. The common sense is really only the first stage, and is the easiest and least labour-intensive. Using experience, knowledge and judgement psychologists generate a large number of questions, from which they will choose a smaller set to be included in the final questionnaire. They choose this sub-set, and make any necessary amendments, based on research. They must establish that the questions make sense, not just to them, but to most, if not all, people. It is very easy for university-educated researchers to make errors in expressing something so that people with less education do not understand them. If a questionnaire is to be useful, it needs to work for most people, rather than for a select few.

Once the researchers have established that the questions make good sense to people, they can start to collect pilot data to look for trends in the way that people answer them. The main reason for this is parsimony. To save time and trouble, both for the researcher and the participant, interviewee or respondent, tests and questionnaires should be as short and as quick-to-complete as possible, without sacrificing sensitivity. If you *must* ask 100 questions to find something out, that is acceptable, but if you can find out just as much (or almost as much) by asking 10, then 90 items should be dropped. When you are ready to take your driving test, you go ahead and take it, rather than spend time and money having more and more lessons when you have reached the examinable standard of driving.

So, psychologists use a representative sample of people to try out the questionnaire or other test. There are many ways of finding a 'representative' sample, just as there are many meanings of the word 'representative'. Just because a set of people seem pretty average does not mean that they are. Do we mean average for the world, or for the country we are in, or for the people we are interested in? Naturally, there are many ways in which the 'average person with diabetes' is not the same as the 'average person'. Without going into detail about sampling methods, suffice to say this is an important part of the research process. Once enough data has been collected psychologists use statistical means to identify the relationships between items on the questionnaire. If the purpose of each item is roughly the same, then what people say in answer to one question should roughly reflect what they say in answer to another. So, one would expect a person who strongly agrees to 'I like to look after my body' to strongly disagree to 'I don't tend to care what happens to my body.' If the relationship was not there, something would probably be amiss. At this stage, researchers identify 'rogue' items, questions which do not cohere with the others. By removing these, they increase the 'togetherness' of the question-naire. In technical language, this is referred to as *internal consistency* or *internal reliability*. If an item is rogue, it adds noise to the data that the scale yields. Listening to what a test tells us can be made more difficult if the results contain noise, just like listening to a radio station can be unpleasant or impossible if the reception is poor.

Once the questionnaire has been streamlined, it can be given to a larger, again representative, sample of people to obtain more information about the test. This tends to come in two ways; data about validity and about reliability.

INTERNAL RELIABILITY (INTERNAL CONSISTENCY)

This is usually determined by Cronbach's alpha (Cronbach, 1951). This is essentially a measure of the relationships (correlations) between items in the scale, producing what one might see as an average correlation between the items in the scale. The higher the value of alpha, the greater the coherence of the scale, and thus the better the internal reliability.

MEASUREMENT SCALES

When you ask someone a question, there are number of ways that you can ask the question, and a number of ways that you can ask someone to answer. You might offer people a YES or NO response, or you might let them write whatever they like in a special box. These represent the two extremes of total restriction of information and complete freedom. The first restricts the answer so much that you might lose valuable information if you forced people to give only one of two responses to each item. (What happens to the people who think 'maybe' or 'it depends on the time and the place'?) The problem with the free-text option is that whilst you are allowing people to say just what they think, you will probably run up against problems when trying to analyse the data. You will find yourself forcing their answers into categories, even when they do not fit, in order to end up with a meaningful analysis. If you leave people to write or say whatever they like in response to a question, the following scenario is possible.

Q: How would you best describe your pain?
A: *It changes from day to day. Sometimes it is like I can taste the pain. Sometimes all of my senses are involved at once.*

If you were trying to analyse this text, you might have problems if you have pre-ordained categories to codify the responses. You might have to decide if this person's answer belongs in one of these categories: strength/weakness, temperature, sharpness/dullness, other. Here some very important information gets lost in the 'other' category, since you have no choice but to put it there. The person did not make reference to the strength of the pain, nor its nature, other than to refer to it in terms of another sensory experience.

Generally, a good compromise between these situations is to adopt some other form of scaling of responses. The most famous type amongst psychologists is the Likert type (Likert, 1952). You will almost certainly have responded to questionnaires with these scales on at some time or other. These involve categories of response, often around five or seven, such as:

strongly agree	agree	neither agree nor disagree	disagree	strongly disagree

It is usual to adopt an odd number of response categories, simply because otherwise it is not possible to allow people to 'sit on the fence' and genuinely not have an opinion or not care one way or another. Such scales must be carefully constructed so that the categories of response mirror each other around the central or neutral point. In order for the scale to make any sense, this symmetry must be in place, so that if one side says 'strongly agree' the other must say 'strongly disagree'.

There is some debate amongst researchers and academics about the appropriate statistical analysis of data derived in this way, but the nature of this is complicated and need not be discussed here. The main issues are simply that one cannot be sure that what 'agree' means to one person is the same as what it means to another. Also we cannot guarantee that the difference between 'agree' and 'strongly agree' is always the same for each person for each item.

Another common scaling method is the visual analogue scale. Here the respondent is presented with a line between two extreme opinions or behaviours and they simply choose and mark a point on the line which shows where they fall between the two. For example:

strongly agree .... **✗**..................... strongly disagree

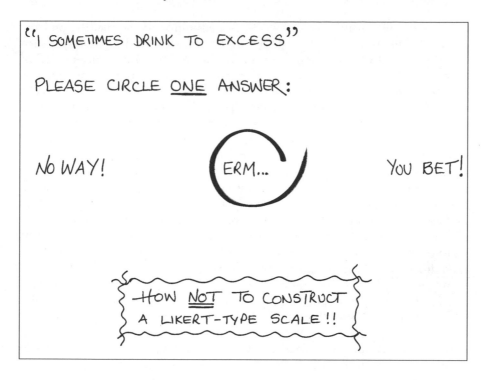

This type of scaling suffers from the same criticisms as the Likert-type scale. Since there is little to discriminate between them, researchers often tend to choose their favourite, or the scale which will be best understood by the respondents. Many articles have been written on scaling methods, and there is still dispute amongst psychologists about what to use and when.

SCALES AND SUB-SCALES

There is another meaning of the term 'scale' that is used by test constructors. Many questionnaires contain more than one type of measurement within them. These are often referred to as sub-scales. An example of this is the Short Form-36 Health Survey (Medical Outcomes Trust, 1993). As the name suggests, there are 36 items which yield, generally, data on a person's general health status from *the person's own perspective*. It consists of eight main sub-scales, including mental health, social and physical functioning, and pain. Scores from the items in each sub-scale are added together before a further mathematical transformation, but the sub-scale scores are not to be added together, because the items are clustered around the themes, and the purpose of the instrument is to gather information on each separately. When questionnaires like this contain sub-scales, they are not necessarily related to each other. If they are independent, then each must be examined individually, as if they were different tests or questionnaires in their own right. Looking at the profile of the scores across sub-scales can, however, give a picture of the respondent's overall status. You would not add together pain and mental health scores to give a composite score, because, after all, what exactly would that number mean? You might, however, say that a person is in moderate pain and experiences some anxiety. You can say that a person has three lemons and a pencil, but not that they have four of anything in particular.

The sub-scales should be researched for their validity and reliability in their own right, once the pilot data has been collected. Internal reliability analysis would only make sense on the sub-scales, not on the questionnaire overall, even though the questionnaire overall is what people filled in.

When a questionnaire contains sub-scales, there is a further statistical analysis which can be applied on the dataset which can pick out the sub-scales and verify them. Factor analysis looks for relationships between answers to questions in a questionnaire and generates 'factors' which are essentially based upon groups of questions. Each question is then given a 'loading', which in simple terms is the extent to which a question or item relates to a factor. Therefore, if there are four sub-scales in a questionnaire, the factor analysis ought to pick out four factors. Hopefully, each question in each sub-scale should load on one factor, and one factor only. When this occurs, the hard work pays off. However, if some questions load on more than one factor, or if there are more or fewer factors than there are sub-scales, something is awry and the designers of the questionnaire must revisit the items and look to create a new scale.

VALIDITY

An important issue is whether the questionnaire or test actually measures what it has been established to measure. This can be very difficult to check on, especially when you are assessing or measuring something you have recently discovered or suggested. You have nothing to compare your data with. This is similar to the situation when radiation was first detected. How could anyone prove that the results of the tests actually showed *radiation* and not something else? (Scientists spend a lot of energy trying to remove the possibility of artefacts spoiling their experiments. Artefacts are things that show up in the data, but are often only there as a by-product of the measurement process, and can be mistaken for the thing being measured itself.) Everything has to be done first by someone, and this can often be a problem because you lack a frame of reference. You can only ever show something in comparison to something else. What is dark without light? What is silence unless you have experienced sound? What is comedy unless you have already been told a joke at some point? Thankfully, many of the things that health psychologists today choose to measure have already been measured, in some form, before. You can establish if your new stress questionnaire really measures people's stress by comparing the results of it with those from existing stress questionnaires. Those questionnaires have, in their turn, been compared with other measures of stress such as blood pressure.

There are quite a number of different types of validity. Only a brief mention of the more common terms is warranted here. For a more thorough discussion of the following, please see books on research methods; recommended are Pelham (1999) and Robson (1993).

Face validity

This is the most basic form of validity, and corresponds to common sense. A test has face validity if, *on the face of it*, it seems to be capable of plucking out the right kind of information. There is nothing technical about face validity.

Construct validity

This is quite a difficult form of validity to define. It is the most important form of validity, and is more philosophical in nature. It essentially revolves around the issue of whether or not what your test is supposed to pick up is a genuine concept that your test really does pick up. Ultimately, this is impossible to demonstrate, since all things can only be measured by measurement items, and are therefore defined by the measurements. For example, there has been substantial argument for decades about the nature of intelligence and what it *really* is. This led to operational definitions being used, which are essentially a sideways step out of the debate. An operational definition is best summed up as a definition of a construct which is inherent in its measurement. Instead of pondering over whether 'health' really exists and if so what exactly it might be, the easy way out is to say that health is something that is demonstrated by health test scores. A healthy person is someone who gets a high score on the test, and a low score defines an unhealthy person. This is a circular argument, admittedly, but allows researchers to get on with the process of measurement and not become bogged down with the theory of knowledge itself.

RELIABILITY

Reliability is the concept relating to the replicability of the results of a test. If we are measuring a stable trait, then if we re-test people we should get the same scores. This is precisely how we test for reliability. A test is reliable if we can give it to people repeatedly (within reason) and achieve the same (or statistically equivalent) scores. If we develop a test for self-esteem, we would expect roughly the same scores from a person on different occasions. Roughly is the right word here, because the reliability of a test is really a concept most determinable when the thing you are testing stays constant over time. People do not tend to suddenly become more intelligent, or the opposite, and so IQ tests do tend to show stable re-test patterns. However, as you will realise, self-esteem is something that can and does alter over time, sometimes in as little as a day or so. This means that if our scores change, it does not mean that the test is not reliable, but perhaps that the self-esteem of the person being tested has changed. Such individual differences cannot be allowed to 'contaminate' the data, which is precisely why large groups of people are needed to determine a test's reliability. Most of the people in a group will not show significant changes in self-esteem over a small period of time. In addition, of those who do, some will show an increase and some a decrease. In a large group, the increases 'cancel out' the decreases, and the steady scores remain. Thus, if we test a large enough and representative enough group of people, most tests should show a good degree of reliability. If they do not, we must ask what is wrong with the test. A well-designed instrument will avoid, for instance, ambiguous items. These can be a source of unreliability. If a question can be interpreted in more than one way, and this can mean a difference in scores depending how the item is interpreted, then this item might be picking up differences in interpretation on re-test, rather than a difference in the thing being measured. If you ask someone the question 'What do you think of the future?' they might legitimately think that this means the future in general, i.e. for people in the world, for the environment, politically and socially, and so on. They might answer based on this interpretation. On another day, they might take this to mean their own personal future. They might be pessimistic about the world's future and optimistic about their own, or vice versa. Thus different answers might be obtained on different occasions. If a person can interpret a question more than one way, then the question is not really picking out any information about the behaviour, phenomenon, ability or trait it was designed to be sensitive to. With experience, we can avoid creating items which may threaten a scale's reliability or validity. If the question above was to be reworded to become 'What do you think about your future?' the problem might be avoided. Another common problem is the double-barrelled question. You should never ask questions like 'Do you think that people who take drugs are sinful and weak-willed?' Does this mean that you have to agree to 'sinful' *and* 'weak-willed' to answer in the affirmative, or only one of them?

It remains to point out that validity and reliability are not entirely discrete concepts. A highly valid questionnaire is likely also to be a reliable one. If you ask enough questions, then averaging across the questions should give you a pretty good measure of what you intend finding out about. Also, the more questions you ask on the right subject, the less chance there is of random fluctuations in the data, that is, the less the chance that someone will give a quirky answer which they would not normally give. If there is little room for the odd quirky answer to affect the data on any given day, then the reliability is higher, and if the questions are asking the right things, there should also be high validity. Imagine that you are a chess expert. Like anyone, you have good and bad days, but on the whole you really are an expert. If you play a novice once, and once only, and you are having a bad day, you might lose when you normally would not. So, if this single match was going to be my test of chess ability, it would not be either reliable *or* valid, because I am unlikely to get the same result on different occasions (reliability) and it is not a good test of chess expertise since it did not pick out the expert from two players (validity). Of course, valid tests are not necessarily *always* reliable, and vice versa.

DOES 'OFF THE SHELF' MEAN GOOD?

People have a tendency to trust off the shelf tests because they have been researched. Students in particular often have considerable faith in the results of their research projects when they have used published tests and inventories. However, 'off the shelf' does not mean 'foolproof', nor should off the shelf tests be used as 'doofers'. According to the old joke, things are called doofers if they will 'do for anything'. Instruments which have been devised for a specific purpose should not be used for other purposes. If a stress inventory has been designed for manual workers, it is likely to be of little use to those wishing to study stress in lawyers. Many questionnaires which purport to be good for general use can present problems for specific populations. Some depression scales are not suitable for certain older people, especially if they detect depression using items which ask things like 'Do you find it difficult to enjoy things which you used to?' Naturally, the normal ageing process can prevent people from enjoying the things they used to. Someone who used to play tennis four times a week may find this difficult when they are in their seventies. In addition, people who are depressed can forget things. So can older people. So a depression scale which asks about memory may fall foul of this problem. Whilst many scales can successfully be used for a range of populations, a good psychologist should work through the items carefully before simply using a test and assuming that it will serve the intended purpose.

USING TESTS

Here are a few key points about using tests, and about developing your own.

- Never add or remove items unless you really must. There are rare occasions when this is necessary, but strictly speaking this should be followed up with further piloting of the new questionnaire and re-collection of normative data. The validity and reliability of a test can, in theory, change dramatically when you remove or add just a single item.
- Never adapt the wording of items unless you really must. For example, if you are intending to give a questionnaire designed for people in general to a group of people with learning disabilities, and no alternative test exists for this population, you will probably need to rephrase items to make them more easily understood. This would be a justifiable case for making changes, although you ought to try and compare the results of both versions on people without learning disabilities to check for validity, and you ought to perform a test like Cronbach's alpha to investigate internal consistency for your adapted instrument. If you have not made significant conceptual changes to the original, then there should not be significant differences between data derived from the two 'versions' of the instrument.
- Respect copyright. Pay for tests where you should, and seek permission to adapt tests from the authors or publishers. Given the tremendous amount of work which goes into the development of tests and questionnaires, using copyrighted material without permission or payment is morally questionable and legally constitutes theft.
- Remember that tests have been devised with specific purposes in mind. You might find that no existing test can help you to find out what you want to. In such cases, making up your own test should be encouraged. In an unresearched area, any measurement tool, however flawed, is better than none, because it starts the ball rolling.

CONCLUDING REMARKS

The next time that you fill in a questionnaire given to you by a reputable market research company, or by a psychologist or other academic researcher or practitioner, try to resist the temptation to think that the time and money taken to produce it was a waste because the questionnaire *looks* as if it had been put together easily. A successful, user-friendly instrument is designed to be simple, clear, obvious and intuitive. However, a lot of work was put in to achieve that. People often say of experts, whether sporting figures or surgeons for instance, that they make what they do 'look easy'. Of course, just because something looks easy does not mean that it is. Unresearched questionnaires should be avoided. Those which have been properly produced and rigorously tested are often relatively costly, and often much more costly than making up your own set of items, but what the cost to you includes is a lot of labour and research which is invaluable in creating a valid, reliable, dependable assessment instrument.

Study questions

1. If you could ask just *one* question to find out how healthy a person was, what would it be?

2. Try to construct a set of questions to measure locus of control. When finished, compare it with an existing locus of control measure.

FURTHER READING

Bowling, A. (1997): *Measuring Health: A review of quality of life measurement scales, Second Edition.* Buckingham: Open University Press.

Bowling, A. (1997): *Research Methods in Health: Investigating Health and Health Services.* Buckingham: Open University Press.

Both books give a good overview of the nature of the issues involved in researching health and in designing scales and other measurement instruments.

9 Chronic Illness, Palliative Care and Death

- Introduction
- Chronic illness
- Palliative care
- Death
- Reacting to death: grief
- Concluding remarks
- Study questions
- Further reading

INTRODUCTION

The concentration of research and writing in health psychology has been on chronic illness. Whilst this is important, chronic illness is often akin to terminal illness in the issues involved (coping, for example). However, in keeping with the medical professions, health psychologists have seemed to shy away from the subject of death and care and support for dying and grieving people. In the last 20 or so years, doctors have realised the folly of this, and have set up a specialism of palliative care medicine. Health psychology must focus more on death and dying. We all will die. We all may need support. It is an irony that the most common event, aside from birth, is death, and yet relatively little research has been directed at understanding it. Perhaps it is a matter of perceived priorities? After all, a dead person needs no care. However, their families and friends do, and they may need considerable support in the time leading up to their death. Palliative care, the support of people who are terminally ill, is aimed specifically at improving quality of life prior to death. The focus is on what *can* be done, not on what cannot. In this sense, health psychologists should be as interested in this as in anything else. Health psychology, in clinical practice, is about maximising health right up until death. It shares this with palliative care.

We begin with a look at chronic illness, and how people adapt and cope with it. Chronic illness, by its nature, is often more about toleration than about cure. We then move to terminal illness, and the process of palliative care. Again, cure is not the essential issue. Finally we examine death as a topic of study for health psychologists. Without an understanding of death, many illness behaviours and cognitions may lack rationale. After all, we should not lose sight of the fact that it is often the perceived threat of death which impels people to give up smoking or take up exercise.

CHRONIC ILLNESS

What is chronic illness? By definition, chronic illness is not something that is easily cured. It is long-lasting, and is usually permanent. It is about a condition which becomes part of a person's life, just as their job or their family is. Anything that makes someone re-evaluate who and what they are has the potential to be a driving factor in their lives. To some people, chronic illness is a part of life which they accept, and to others it is a devastating thing which makes their lives feel less valuable. Which reaction occurs depends upon the personality of the individual, the support they require and whether it is matched by that which they receive, and the severity of the illness. Common chronic illnesses include diabetes, arthritis, heart disease, asthma and Crohn's disease (affecting the digestive tract).

Upon diagnosis, Shontz (1975) describes a set of stages through which people may seem to pass. Initially there is **shock**, upon hearing the diagnosis. This is considerably more profound when the diagnosis was entirely unexpected, for example when a person with a persistent thirst but no other symptoms is told that they have diabetes. Following this, the patient may undergo an **encounter reaction**, involving many negative feelings, distress, and possibly anger. The third phase, known as **retreat**, is essentially denial, where the patient acts as if the disease or illness is simply not present, is not happening to them. Eventually the patient leaves these stages and comes to terms with the illness. These are not set in stone. Some people will not show any reaction which is clearly classifiable as one of these in isolation, others show a blend of them at any one time. Later you will read about Kübler-Ross's (1969) stages in response to a diagnosis of terminal illness, and the similarities are marked.

A common reaction to a diagnosis is to ascribe blame, often self-blame. In many illnesses, people look for a reason why they have succumbed to it. People will look to environmental exposures or to their own lack of self-care. They may lay the blame at the door of those around them. There is a very mixed literature on this issue: some researchers claim that self-blame is harmful to the individual, some that it is a coping strategy with positive aspects to it, and others that it has little effect on anything. As research progresses, we may be able to identify individuals for whom self-blame may be positive and for whom it may be negative, with a view to modifying such a perception of causation. An example of self-blame working for the good of an individual comes from

Hampson (1997). She showed that self-blame is a common causative explanation of diabetes, and that diabetics who self-blame are often those who demonstrate greatest control over their illness. This makes some sense; if a person thinks that their behaviours have caused their illness, they ought also to believe that they are capable of controlling it themselves and managing it too.

Social comparison

A key coping mechanism which has been identified in chronic illness, which sets it apart from coping with terminal illness, is social comparison. Dealt with by, amongst others, Taylor (1983), this is a term to describe the reaction of viewing the diagnosis and prognosis of chronic illness as interpretable only in comparison with other people experiencing hardship in life. Indeed, this is a form of coping based upon re-evaluation of the state of affairs. You have probably known people who have said things like:

- 'Mustn't complain too much . . . there are people who are worse off . . .'
- 'It could have been worse . . . . like that poor woman down the road . . .'
- 'At least I am not dying . . .'
- 'My uncle had such a hard life . . . compared to me, that is . . .'

These are examples of social comparison coping. Taylor *et al* (1984) looked at coping mechanisms in women who had been diagnosed with breast cancer. They improved their perceptions of their illness by a process of downward comparison. This means that they adapted to their situation by looking for examples of people who were worse off than them. Of course, social comparison can also be a negative force. If a person is genuinely worse off than those around them, or, more importantly, if they perceive themselves to be worse off than others, then this is not a constructive coping mechanism, since the person is likely to feel struck by fate or annoyed at their 'bad luck'.

Diabetes

An example of chronic illness which is common is diabetes. Most people know someone who is diabetic, to a greater or lesser degree. The hormone insulin, secreted by the pancreas, controls the levels of glucose (a sugar) present in the blood. When this system goes wrong, diabetes results. Too much sugar in the blood is called hyperglycaemia, and this leads to **diabetes mellitus**. There are two main forms of this, insulin-dependent, and non-insulin-dependent, also called Type I and Type II. The former is much rarer than the latter, making up no more than a tenth of cases of diabetes. In insulin-dependent diabetes mellitus, people must inject themselves with insulin in order to maintain their blood sugar levels, usually because the insulin-producing cells in the pancreas are physically or chemically damaged and unable to function. This type tends to develop early in life. In Type II diabetes injections are not necessary because the cells in the pancreas can still produce insulin and so regulation of blood sugar is achieved by giving nature a 'helping hand'. Quite simply, by careful regulation of diet and taking of medication the problem can be kept under control. This type of diabetes is most likely to develop at middle-age, although it can occur at any age.

Diabetes is not just a health problem in itself. It is accompanied by a set of risk factors for other life-threatening conditions, and it can have effects on the life of an individual over and above the challenges faced by daily injections or by being careful about food. People with diabetes are more likely to fall prey to strokes, heart attacks, develop kidney disease, become blind, and, in men, develop erectile dysfunction. Diabetes is also a secondary complication in a number of other conditions, such as cystic fibrosis and liver cirrhosis. It is one of the most common diseases, affecting 30 million people worldwide (Gale and Anderson, 1998).

The ordinary lives of people coping with diabetes were described by the sociologist Kelleher (1988). In interviews with 30 diabetics from London, he identified three life strategies. The 'true' copers were those who fitted diabetes into their lives without changing their lifestyle significantly, and followed doctors' advice. These people (20% of the sample) showed a high degree of personal control, something deemed very important by health psychologists studying chronic illness. They were in charge of their illness, rather than it being in charge of them. Thirty per cent of the interviewees showed what Kelleher calls an adaptive strategy. These people make changes to their lifestyle, but lack some of the control that the copers do. They normalised their diabetes, accepting it as part of their life. Their lives changed more as a result of coping with diabetes than the true copers. Finally, the most important group in some sense was the worriers, who comprised a half of the sample. These people dealt with their illness by worrying about it continually. They tended not to be able to see diabetes as a part of their normal life, and generally rated themselves as unhealthy people, diabetes being something, to them, which *per se* makes them unhealthy. Depression and anxiety characterised these people. An important distinction between the first two groups and the last is that the latter would see themselves as primarily a diabetic, rather than as a person with social roles and a place in the world. The others saw their diabetes as secondary, rather than primary. This is the difference between what we might call a diabetic man, and a man with diabetes, or a diabetic woman with two children or a mother of two who has diabetes. By identifying this core perception, health psychologists ought to be able to work with a person to find the most suitable path through the career of the illness.

Unlike some other chronic illnesses which may rely mainly upon management of the condition by doctors using drugs and equipment, the progress of diabetes depends upon a great deal of self-management. Not everyone is equipped with the skills to be able to do this naturally. Just as there are people with tidy offices and untidy offices, or people who make good use of their time and people who 'waste' it, so there are people who are able to take control over their life to make the changes necessary to keep diabetes in check, and there are those who find the changes in diet and lifestyle tremendously stressful. Getting people to stick to a controlled lifestyle is often very difficult, especially amongst certain groups, such as diabetic adolescents, who often feel that diabetes is preventing them from being just like their friends and taking part in everything they do. Furthermore, many of the dangers inherent in failing to follow self-care and self-treatment regimes (controlling diet and so on) are not immediate ones. Therefore, people are not scared by failing to look after themselves in an ideal fashion, because they may not notice any physical changes whatsoever: some of the problems of mismanaged diabetes will not occur for decades. The threat of a problem in 30 years time is not a strong one to most people.

Insulin-dependent diabetics have to make calculations to determine how much insulin to inject. This is because there are a number of factors which affect how much is needed, such as exercise and stress. Therefore, rather than a set dosage, insulin requirements have to be tested using a sample of blood. If a person makes the wrong dosage choice, the result could be fatal, especially if the individual repeatedly misinjects themselves over a sustained period.

It is often said that knowledge is power. Of course, power is also about control. Can knowledge affect control? It appears so, but not necessarily linearly. Hamburg and Inoff (1982) studied children and adolescent diabetic people attending a summer camp set up specifically for them. Dividing them into three groups, those who knew little about their illness, those who knew a fair amount, and those who knew a considerable amount, proved very telling. On a measure of adherence, that is the extent to which the diabetic adolescents went along with doctors' advice on treatment, the relatively ignorant group showed poorer adherence than those with a moderate amount of knowledge. However, the lowest rates of adherence were found in the young people who knew the most about diabetes. This led the authors to suggest that the reality of the seriousness of diabetes can be debilitating and depressing for those people who know most about what their bodies are doing, and are fully aware of the 'life sentence' of chronic illness. Whilst the phrase 'ignorance is bliss' seems inappropriate here, too much knowledge can bring a degree of *disempowerment* and reduce control.

Langewitz *et al* (1997) report an educational and problem-solving programme intended to improve self-management in diabetic people. The participants were involved in both experiential learning of the effects of various factors upon blood glucose levels and also worked through 'solutions' to problems about dosages. The programme significantly improved blood glucose levels, and reduced diabetes-related illness, showing that self-management is a skill which can be developed substantially.

As with other chronic illnesses, the stress that diabetes can engender in an individual must be appropriately managed in order to prevent it creating additional health problems. Since diabetes is associated with poorer cardio-vascular health, stress can exacerbate this because stress itself, as we have seen elsewhere, is also a factor in heart disease. However, there is by no means a simple relationship between stress reduction and health in diabetic patients. Alkens et al (1997) compared non-insulin-dependent diabetics assigned to either a stress-reducing muscle-relaxation and imagery programme or to standard medical treatment. Blood glucose levels were tested before and after the programme, and 16 weeks after the intervention. They found that blood glucose levels could actually be lowered by the muscle-relaxation programme, but principally in the group of people who were less stressed to begin with. This suggests that, as with virtually any treatment programme, medical or otherwise, there will be individual differences in the reaction to it and its effectiveness. Health psychologists are actively involved in the quest to discover what those individual differences are, with the aim of tailoring therapeutic interventions appropriately.

Cancer

Cancer (neoplasm) is the development of abnormal cells in the body. It can occur in any tissue, including bone or blood cells. It can be benign, which means that it is relatively harmless and will not spread, or malignant. Malignant neoplasms are prone to spreading by cells leaving the tumour and moving elsewhere in the body (known as metastasis). Cancer is another major issue in the study of chronic illness. It affects about a third of us, eventually. It is an interesting disease since it bridges the gap between chronic illness and palliative care. Not all people with cancer die from it by any means. When cancer is not decidedly terminal, it is often essentially a chronic illness, since it may take years to be treated successfully. Freud himself, for instance, spent many years struggling against cancer in the latter part of his life. However, when cancer defeats the doctors and the patients, it is then a case for palliative care.

Cancer is an emotive issue, especially since it affects so many people. Most of us know someone who has died of cancer, and many of us will know people who have had cancer but have survived it. It is an emotive subject not just for patients, but for their families and their doctors and nurses. Wilkinson (1991) examined the issue of how nurses communicate with cancer patients. The communication styles used by nurses were classified into four categories. Some nurses were facilitators. They were largely able to help patients to express their fears and concerns, and to deal with issues successfully. They picked up on cues from the patients that they were needing to talk, and responded to them appropriately. Others were ignorers. They chose to avoid patients' cues, getting on with other things rather than being drawn into conversations about their feelings. Another group were the informers. They dealt mainly with the 'facts' about the patients' cases, providing information but little more. Their focus was on the concrete situation, rather than the more abstract. Mixers were nurses who had facilitative skills, but who also used a blocking strategy at times to prevent patients from raising difficult issues. This blocking strategy was found in most nurses. Rather than always deal with what a patient seems to need to talk about, they would often divert attention away from this. Why this occurs is understandable, but it is far from ideal. The emotional drain on nurses caused by dealing with patients' feelings is damaging to their own health, at least in principle, and with limited resources nurses are simply prioritising. This is a good example of where a health psychologist or counsellor can be of use in health services. Since nurses may lack communication skills in these cases, and lack time, there is an argument for using the skills of other professionals to fill the gap.

What, then, do cancer patients feel? They experience a range of emotions, as one would expect, and their histories and personalities will affect these. There is some evidence, also, to show that the course of their illness interacts with their emotions and cognitions. Some research has suggested that there is a **Type C personality**. Just as there has been work directed at identifying types of people who are most likely to develop heart disease (the Type A/Type B distinction), there is also some evidence that some people are more prone to develop cancer than others, the so-called Type C personality (Temoshok, 1987). The Type C person tends to repress their emotions rather than give vent to them. In this respect, they are the opposite of the Type A person. They do not tend to express anger, they do not forgive others easily, but they work hard to fit in with others and give in to their requirements. They are co-operative, even when their own needs conflict with those of others. Some have suggested that they indulge in self-pity more than average, that they lack social support networks because they tend to be loners, and that they often have a poor self-image. Many psychologists are sceptical about the cancer-predisposing personality, but a study by Shaffer et al (1987) suggests that there is such a thing. Almost 1000 doctors were tracked over three decades, and those who gave vent to their feelings were 16 times less likely to develop cancer than those who 'bottled up' their feelings. This study did not suffer from a flaw which has dogged research into personality and health in general. Many studies look at people after they have developed an illness, assess their personalities, and then compare them to a control group. Of course, illness can change personality. The only good way to approach this particular topic is to assess a large number of people, and then to wait until they become ill during the natural course of their life, looking for trends in disposition and disease developed. This is what Shaffer et al (1987) did.

Some theorists suggest that the personality–cancer link works through psychoneuroimmunology. Basically, holding in one's feelings causes stress, and stress suppresses the immune system. A suppressed immune system is less able to deal with the rogue cells which develop in our bodies quite regularly. When the rogue cells are not dealt with, they proliferate and become the disease cancer.

Treatments for cancer are themselves the source of a great deal of stress for patients. They are rarely effected rapidly, usually taking months or years. They involve intense nausea, weakness, and loss of hair (essentially signs of radiation sickness, since radiation is used to treat cancer, even though it is one of its causes). Patients can, therefore, fall prey to feelings of cognitive dissonance. They are being cared for and treated by doctors, but actually feel much worse than when they were not. At times, it can be difficult for them to believe that the additional pain caused by the treatment is worth it. Since the treatment causes nausea, they can often start to develop a conditioned response. As a result, various factors in their environment start to make them feel ill just because they associate them with the treatment (Jacobsen *et al*, 1993). However, people do expect treatments to have side effects, especially those for cancer about which they may have heard a great deal. Leventhal *et al* (1986) found that women with breast cancer were anxious about their chemotherapy because it did not have significant side effects. They equated this with a lack of powerfulness of the treatment, and were concerned that they were not having their cancer treated with the most potent therapy available.

Cancer presents an unusual post-treatment threat, since unlike other illnesses or diseases there is always a concern that it might return, only for the patient to have to undergo anxiety-provoking tests and treatments all over again. There is evidence to show that the psychological distress caused from a diagnosis of recurrent cancer is greater than that generated from the original diagnosis.

Research into coping with cancer has found that 'fighting spirit' is important, which is explained later in this chapter. For some people, denial is an effective strategy. Pettingale *et al* (1985) found a survival advantage of five to ten years in breast cancer patients who denied or fought their illness after diagnosis. As Salmon (2000) asserts, however, the relationship between a coping strategy and survival is a correlational one, which does not necessarily imply direct causation. Other factors might pin together these two. For instance, fighting spirit can lead to better nursing care, which leads to better survival. If you are a 'fighter', the staff may like you more. You might eat more, to help you fight the disease. Or, a predisposition to surviving cancer might be provided by a gene which is also linked to having a fighting-spirit personality. However, as Dunkel-Schetter *et al* (1992) found, over a half of patients with cancer did not have a main coping strategy. We might think, at first, that this is a bad thing, but we must remember that a person who does not have a main coping strategy may use a mixture of strategies to cope, and is perhaps better off than someone who relies on one strategy for all eventualities. Those 'mixers' amongst us may be the most adaptive people who, in some circumstances, might be the best equipped to tackle problems and threats.

We are only just beginning to understand how psychologically complicated cancer is, and so we are a long way from understanding its entire psychosocial effects. People's health behaviours can be affected by fears of cancer, and people who develop cancer have a range of reactions to it, and to the diagnosis, the prognosis, the treatment, and the risk of recurrence. All of these may be affected by psychosocial mechanisms. Since cancer is such a prevalent disease, the future of health psychology will be one where it figures heavily in research.

Control

Without entering into considerable detail, it is necessary to point out that much of what has been said about chronic illness centres around the issue of control. Generally, patients who feel in control of their illness cope better than those who feel, in contrast, that they are somehow at the mercy of it. Fighting spirit cannot exist without some sense of personal control, and many other coping strategies rely upon the individual keeping a tight rein on their own thoughts and behaviours. Self-management of treatment regimes is achieved more easily when a person believes that doing so is within their grasp. However, control is not always a good thing. Pain relief, used for many chronic illnesses such as cancer or arthritis, can be handed over to the patient. This is known as patient-controlled analgesia (PCA), and can involve administering direct injections of painkillers into a vein via a machine which the patient controls. This not only gives the patient a hand in managing their own symptoms, but also frees up the time of the health professionals, who would otherwise have to administer the analgesia. Research indicates that control is not always the important issue, but simply gaining access to pain relief when it is required. Since doctors and nurses are not always available, patients suffer until they are. PCA prevents this occurring, since when pain relief is needed, pain relief is available. Patients do not seem to care *who* does the job, as long as it is done (Taylor *et al*, 1996).

Control can take a number of forms. Taylor *et al* (1984) looked at the relationship between control and adjustment to breast cancer, comparing a number of types of control. Cognitive control seemed to be associated with the most adjustment, which is thinking about the cancer and life differently and 'filing away' negative ideas in a neat fashion. Interestingly, there was no relationship between adjustment to breast cancer and informational control. This means that having knowledge about breast cancer from information leaflets and the like did not assist the women in coming to terms with their disease. This suggests that information can, at times, simply increase fear, especially reading about the probabilities of your own death, or treatments which involve a lot of discomfort.

PALLIATIVE CARE

Palliative care is the support provided for people who are terminally ill. They represent a challenging group to doctors, since they are a reminder of the failures of medicine. Medicine is seen as a largely curative phenomenon, and terminally ill people are those whom medicine cannot help. Palliative care, historically, has been a non-medical aspect of healthcare. It had been, until relatively recently, an issue for charities to deal with, and many people working with terminally ill people were volunteers. Of course, this approach was not satisfactory. To leave their care to kind helpers is to play down the needs of dying people. There is no reason, other than a financial one, why dying people should be dealt with in any way differently from other patients or clients in a healthcare system.

Whilst palliative care is, in the public eye, all about death, nothing could be further from the truth. It is best defined by what it is not: it is not all about death and dying. Palliative care shares the same values of standard curative care: looking after people, supporting them, and providing the best possible quality of life until life is over. Since every person dies, there is no difference between the ethos underpinning curative care and that underpinning palliative care. Palliative care is about life, not death, and comfort, not grief. It is important to note that, almost without exception, palliative care worldwide is focused on life rather than death, and so euthanasia (the ending of life by medical means to relieve suffering) is not perceived as a branch of it. The ethos is usually about relieving suffering in a living being, rather than relieving suffering by ending life.

Palliative care is unusual in that the contribution of non-medical professionals is seen as invaluable. In fact, the relative contributions are reversed. Usually, doctors take precedence over psychologists and the like. However, in the case of palliative care, doctors' power is considerably less, since they are not able to cure the patients. The emphasis is on quality of life, something which psychologists can make significant enhancements to. Indeed, in palliative care the psychologist, doctor, and comedy entertainer can all make equivalent contributions.

Psychological contributions to the study of the palliative care process have focused around two issues, namely reaction to the diagnosis and prognosis, and improvement of the quality of remaining life. Kübler-Ross (1969) was amongst the first to systematically set out the stages of reaction to a diagnosis of terminal illness. In her work there are five stages, which are not rigidly determined: one does not have to experience all of them, although the most common pattern is to do so, in the order outlined.

- **Stage one – denial:** In this stage, the individual has difficulty believing the diagnosis. They refuse to accept that it is happening to them. This refusal can take the form of questioning the diagnosis or, in more extreme cases, either refusing to talk about the issue and carrying on as normal, or simply flatly denying the fact of the diagnosis. In its purest form, denial is quite a shocking reaction, since it is tantamount to refuting the knowledge of one's senses.

- **Stage two – anger:** In this stage, the individual begins to vent anger. A diagnosis of terminal illness can cause a person to lash out at those who made the diagnosis, or indeed anyone involved. It is not uncommon for the person to be insulting to those who are supporting them, even to blame them for the problem. Essentially, the anger is generally based around feelings of injustice, that is, it is simply not fair that it has happened to them.
- **Stage three – bargaining:** The manifestation of this phase can depend upon spirituality, since the bargains made here are often with a divine power. The dying person may ask their god for strength to remain alive until the end of the year, or the month, or until a friend gets married, and so on. There is some degree of acceptance of the inevitability of death, but also a feeling that something can be done to change the facts and events surrounding it.
- **Stage four – depression:** Possibly the most difficult stage, here a depression takes hold because the body and mind are more and more fatigued and the reality of the impending end becomes clearer and closer. With less and less time left, the person has fewer things to look forward to. Depression is therefore, a natural outcome.
- **Stage five – acceptance:** Finally, the person comes to terms with their illness and with death itself. They cease fighting it, and they allow it to take its course. In many ways, they are often now too weak to do anything other than submit to 'fate' and to nature. The extent to which the acceptance is genuine and to which it is forced upon the individual due to a lack of resources is debatable. Sometimes the acceptance is very philosophical in nature, where the dying person sees the process as providing closure, and at other times it may seem to be a form of learned helplessness, where a person simply gives in and gives up.

There is little scientific support for these as stages *per se*. Many people experience just one of these reactions and stick with it, whereas others vacillate between all of them, and at times seem to blend them together. What is important about the typology put forward by Kübler-Ross is that we have a description of the *range* of reactions. Most reactions to a diagnosis of terminal illness involve one or more of these, and they rarely involve anything else.

Kastenbaum has devoted most of his career to developing a psychological understanding of death. Kastenbaum (2000) puts forward no less than 17 models of reactions to death, most of which have consequences for the health and well-being of the dying individual. Whilst they are not models in the sense in which psychologists usually use the term, they give an insight into the vast range of thoughts which occupy a person who is terminally ill. To summarise, but hopefully to retain a flavour of Kastenbaum's models, he suggests that dying people:

- may view themselves as facing dwindling physical and mental resources
- may experience a distorted body image since parts of it may change as a result of illness, and may also have a sense of cognitive malfunctioning or 'madness'
- may view themselves as contagious and could pass death on to others
- feel that they have lost their status and power as an individual
- may feel that others do not take them seriously
- may feel without a coping strategy, since one only ever dies once and cannot be 'prepared'
- may distort time and can focus on not having enough time left to achieve things
- feel that they are losing everything they have, including the love of others
- may become detached from the world because attachment seems futile
- feel that they are on a journey
- feel that they are closing a book which cannot be re-opened
- feel that they are 'performing' in a tragic play and wish to be seen as a good performer, and that their life is a story which they must seek meaning in.

As health psychologists, we can attach some of these models to our own models of health and illness behaviour. Some of the above are associated with control factors, others with learned helplessness, and so on. One thing that strikes us clearly from this list is that death is like no other aspect of health psychology in that it happens only once. People become ill regularly throughout their lives, and much of what health psychologists have to offer is applicable at all times. Death is something which, it seems, we must research, but our findings will only be of use to each person once.

The issue of hope

A key factor in palliative care work is that of hope. It may seem odd to speak of hope in patients for whom there is no hope, as it were. This is true, and the central problem facing palliative care professionals is dismantling hope. For reasons such as denial, patients may simply continue to have overly optimistic thoughts about the prognosis of their illness. They may believe that a cure will be found tomorrow, or that they will miraculously get better despite what the doctors have told them. Whilst such things can and do occur, they are extremely rare, and most diagnoses of terminal illness are accurate. Taking away a person's hope can be a very important issue, because to an extent people need to realise the truth about their situation, in order that they can come to terms with it properly and make suitable plans.

False hope is common and, as Nekolaichuk and Bruera (1998) point out, there are three popular myths which may underpin forms of hope. The first is the myth of 'immortality', whereby we generally live our lives without contemplating the only real certainty in it, that of our death. This carries over into the palliative care setting, with patients simply refusing to believe that they could be dying. The second myth is that of the 'magic bullet'. This is the belief that patients have that they will die quickly and painlessly, and that doctors can help them to die in this way. Not only are doctors forbidden by law from doing this (except in the Netherlands, where, at the time of writing, laws are being changed to allow euthanasia), but they often lack the tools to be able to bring about a peaceful end. The third myth named is that of 'truth telling'. Patients may believe that what they have been told about their condition is the truth and that it is all that there is to know. There is, of course, at times, a large discrepancy between what a doctor tells a patient and what is really happening, especially important when the doctor believes that knowing the truth will deleteriously affect the quality of life of a patient.

Finally, Hinton (1999) has shown that, in cancer patients, psychological distress interacts with prognosis in interesting ways. Whilst people do seem to come to accept a prognosis of terminal illness over time, this can waver as death becomes nearer. In addition, anxiety is greater when a patient is told that death is probable than when they are told that it is certain. Therefore, a doctor who seeks to provide hope by 'leaving the door open' for a patient and saying that they will probably die could be creating more anxiety than one who says that they will.

The meaning of dying

Different cultures perceive the process of dying in different ways, something which those working in palliative care need to be aware of. There is not one, single, fixed meaning of death, and there is not one, single, fixed pathway to it. It is easy to be ignorant of cultural issues surrounding death, and it is just as easy to be insensitive as a result.

Payne *et al* (1996) examined the meaning of a 'good death' amongst dying patients and health professionals. There was a mismatch found. They interviewed 18 patients and 20 health professionals, and discovered that what patients tend to see as a good death is one where there is no pain, dying quickly, and often with no consciousness, such as dying during sleep. The issue of a dignified death was also raised. However, the health professionals focused on the control of symptoms, absence of distress, and the involvement of family. Whilst some of these themes overlap, there is a distinct difference in the way in which the two groups conceptualise death. What this shows us, of course, is that we must be careful to be aware that what we feel is not necessarily what others will feel, something which is especially important when medical professionals are aiming to provide the best care for a person. Putting in place what you think a person wants is not necessarily bound to achieve the aim of fulfilling the person's wishes.

Foley *et al* (1995) have showed that AIDS presented a culturally-based challenge to palliative care previously unfaced. In their study, based in Canada, a large proportion of people dying from AIDS-related illnesses were gay men. Most palliative care, statistically, is directed at older people, usually with children, wider families, and partners. The older you get, the greater the chance that you will die of a terminal illness. In addition, most palliative care services are used by people with forms of malignant neoplasm (commonly known as cancer). In fact, as Eve *et al* (1997) state, less than 4% of referrals in the UK to palliative care are for diseases other than cancer. People with AIDS do not tend to fit the pattern, and less so if they are gay. They may be ostracised from their social circle or family, on account of having AIDS, which is still a heavily stigmatised illness. Generally, people do not pass moral judgement on people dying from cancer or the like. They do not tend to blame them for their illness, and do not tend to see their illness as a punishment for their behaviour. AIDS is not like this. Because for many people it is erroneously associated with gay lifestyles, and because gay lifestyles are often frowned upon, gay people with AIDS are generally given less sympathy and support. We have seen elsewhere in this book the importance of social support in determining the course of an illness. Some people with AIDS may have already lost friends or partners in this way, and so are very aware of the course of their illness, which may create considerable anxiety. Multiple bereavements are not uncommon in this population, adding to the grief with every new diagnosis (Cho and Cassidy, 1994). There are additional stresses, such as the fact that many insurers will not pay sickness or death benefits for people with AIDS who have acquired HIV sexually. Furthermore, many gay men never have children. As a result, they often do not have the comfort found by many straight people: that their children will remain after their death and their family name or genes will be carried on. For many people this is a great source of hope for the future. All of this means that the counselling and support offered to such patients must be substantially different from that provided to the 'average' palliative care patient.

If we look at culture in the more conventional sense, then the needs which arise for different groups can be extremely diverse. Sometimes they may conflict with other clinical concerns and other cultures. Patients in palliative care wards are often together, rather than in separate rooms, especially so in non-private healthcare systems such as the British National Health Service. Sikhs and Hindus both traditionally die with family around them, and religious chanting around the dying person is usual (Firth, 2000). Of course, to people who do not share these values, this may seem a disruption to other patients. It may frighten other patients who are not familiar with this behaviour and who may be only semi-conscious because of analgesic drugs which have psychoactive effects. Clearly what is required is some way of providing for all patients and their families. It is no more right to tell the family of a dying Sikh that they must refrain from chanting than it is for the non-Sikh patient to listen to the chanting if it alarms them. As more cultural awareness seeps into societies, so hospitals can make appropriate moves to try to please all people most of the time. Many Hindus prefer to die on the floor, and so will make efforts to lie on the floor should they feel as if they are about to pass away. However, there have been anecdotal reports of nurses, unaware of this tradition, forcing patients to return to bed. Again, a little cultural awareness can prevent a great deal of distress in a case such as this.

Little is known about ethnicity and responses to dying and death. Most of the research conducted has been on the historically 'standard' patient: usually white, usually heterosexual, usually of Christian social origin. The classic work on understanding death, reactions to terminal illness, and bereavement and grief, has been based upon data from such populations. The future for palliative care, and the involvement of health psychologists in it, must be one of inclusiveness. If we want to appreciate the diversity of human health behaviour, we must explore all, not some, of it.

One serious gap in the investigations into the meaning of terminal illness has been that of sexuality. As outlined above, AIDS itself was a new challenge to palliative care providers. However, as Gilley (2000) points out, there are virtually no mentions of sexuality *per se* in the palliative care literature. Dying people seem to be regarded as asexual, with little or no interest in sexual behaviour. This, of course, may be very true when people are too weak to move or are in intense pain. But for many other people sexual gratification, and intimacy, may be an important factor in determining quality of life. It may be an affirmation of love and of the fact that they are still alive. It can be seen as a form of esteem support. Appropriate sexual counselling and encouragement may be necessary, but palliative care workers need to be aware of the sexual needs of their clients. As health psychologists become more valued and involved in such cases, so we may develop a greater awareness of the issues surrounding terminal illness and sexual behaviour.

Informal palliative care

Many people who are dying prefer to do so at home, away from the hospital environment. Since palliative care resources are limited, and since the patient has requested this, doctors are keen to support such a strategy as long as it is not clinically obstructive, that is it does not mean that the patient will receive less effective care. Whilst this move to the home environment has its advantages, there is also a burden placed upon the carer or carers which needs to be recognised. Health psychology should not just be about health and disease in people themselves, but about the impact of health behaviours or illness on those around the individual. Research has shown that considerable stress is placed upon the carer (usually a partner or family member) when a dying person chooses to spend their remaining life at home. Payne *et al* (1999), in a study of 39 informal carers, reported that 84% of them were under additional stress and 41% seemed to be undergoing rather high levels of stress. What this means is that whilst the patient is being cared for in the best way for them, the carer is risking their own health, both mental and physical. As Grande *et al* (1997) found, this may lead the carers to ask for more help from external agencies such as the community health services, but doing so can be contrary to the patient's wishes, causing additional concern. Also, patients themselves often feel like they would prefer to be independent but are in need of support, thus threatening independence. Both situations are examples of **cognitive dissonance,** as described by Festinger (1957). When two outcomes are needed, but one interferes with the other, the strain produced can be detrimental to health.

Some of the stress associated with the process of dying and of palliative care is expressed by de Montigny (1993). It seems that, as a coping mechanism, silence is used by both patients and their carers. It is not unusual to find scenes where no-one is talking, and de Montigny points out that these are very pregnant silences, rather than meaningless ones. Since cognitive dissonance is about irresolvable contradiction, it is not surprising that people often adopt silence. With no satisfactory answer likely, there is, it is perceived, no reason to ask a question. What this author suggests is that a great deal of information about the state of mind of the patient and caregiver can be gleaned from ordinary utterances, rather than from direct talk about death itself. Sometimes, psychologists must be indirect in their methods, especially when sensitive and painful issues are being aired.

Defeating terminal illness

There are documented cases of people surviving a diagnosis of terminal illness. These may represent a good opportunity for health psychologists to examine the power that the mind has over the bodily mechanisms. Greer (1991) identified a survival characteristic associated with the coping style first referred to by Derogatis *et al* (1979): 'fighting spirit'. In a 15-year study, 62 women were followed up after a diagnosis of breast cancer. Five reactions were identified: fighting spirit, stoic acceptance, helplessness/hopelessness, anxious preoccupation and denial. Denial needs no explanation. Anxious pre-occupation is a greater-than-normal level of worry and focus on the cancer. Helplessness/hopelessness is exactly what it sounds like. Stoic acceptance is taking a philosophical stance, almost like that of the existentialist philosophers, taking on board the diagnosis as part of life and accepting it, since it is what it is. Those with fighting spirit are the people who accept the diagnosis, but refuse to let cancer 'beat them'. They fight the illness, using all of their resources. After 15 years, almost a half of the women who were characterised by their fighting spirit were alive, compared with less than a fifth in the other coping-style groups. This seems to suggest that fighting an illness, which is largely a psychological response, pays dividends. Without entering into details here, the research into fighting spirit, however, remains balanced; studies both for and against its protective effect exist.

DEATH

To say that people differ in their reactions to, and beliefs about, death is to state the obvious. One might say that death is of crucial interest to health psychologists. When people develop health behaviours, might they do so because they fear death? When people develop health cognitions and values, might they not be shaped by fear of the worst consequence of ill health: death?

The study of death is generally called thanatology. When Freud (largely ignored by psychologists today) first described an innate desire to self-destruct, he called this thanatos, the death instinct. According to psychoanalytic theory, human beings have two competing drives: the life instinct and the death instinct. Psychoanalysts can use the concept of a death instinct to explain self-harming behaviour, and our fascination with death, either in movies or in real life. Whilst Freud has little place in modern health psychology, the thanatos does have some common sense validity, and can be useful in understanding, perhaps, why people engage in life-threatening behaviours. Willis (1993) describes the significance of death as a concept in 'biker' culture. To these motorcyclists, death is something to be fought with. They frequently have encounters with death because of the nature of their interest, which is, ultimately, a relatively dangerous one. Willis points out that they do not have an obvious death-wish, but that they enjoy the threat of death as the vehicle for a challenge to survive. In many ways, these people may be likened to any other people who take risks, such as smokers.

REACTING TO DEATH: GRIEF

We tend to use the term 'grief' to describe a particular reaction and set of coping mechanisms, that is the reaction to a death. In fact, one can grieve over any loss. It does not have to be a death, as such. So, it is legitimate to use the term to describe the reaction to loss of an arm, or the loss of one's sight. However, we will concentrate here on grief in its most obvious and commonly used sense.

Grief depends upon many things. Who dies, and who lives to grieve, is a key factor. Although it is difficult to generalise from situation to situation, personal circumstance to personal circumstance, it is probably fair to say that losing a child is different from losing a parent. One is statistically more likely than the other, and, as a result, may be easier to deal with. The natural order is for older people to die before younger ones, and people expect this. But, whoever dies there is likely to be stress and trauma.

Grief is a socially constructed phenomenon as much as it is an individual one. Through social norms, cultural values, friends, family, religious leaders and the media we are shown how to behave when someone dies and what to do. We hear of people saying that someone had a 'good send-off' or a 'fitting tribute', and we also hear of 'tasteless' treatments of death. What this means is that the process of grief and the outward signs of it are tempered by what others expect of us. In some cultures people are expected to publicly display their grief by openly crying or wailing and by wearing black, or some other colour of clothing, sometimes for prescribed periods of time. In other cultures death is welcomed and must not be mourned. Displaying 'appropriate' grief has been mulled over by Walter *et al* (2000). They suggest that experts on grief have suggested three contradictory hypotheses about the culture of grief in Britain. The first is that traditional mourning rituals developed by the Victorians have dissipated, leaving people with no guide as to how to behave. This is why some people report not knowing what to say to people who are bereaved. The second hypothesis is that there are cultural norms within mainstream British culture, but that they are implicit rather than explicit, leading to confusion. There is an expectancy that a person will display moderate signs of grief, but remain tough and maintain their resolve despite the trauma. This 'stiff upper lip' which, it is suggested, is typical of British behaviour, can backfire. If a person fails to show *enough* grief-related behaviour, they are thought of as callous and their concern for the deceased could be called into question. The third hypothesis, a development of this, states that extreme grief and anxiety is permissible socially, but with constraints as to when and where it should happen. It is acceptable to be distraught at home, but not amongst strangers in public. The suggestion is that this could cause problems because the strangers will not know why the person is crying. Of course, this relates to the first hypothesis, that we have lost some of our rituals of grief. A hundred years ago, a woman who lost her husband would wear all black clothing, and often a black veil, for quite some time after the death. A man would usually wear a black armband for a period of time after the death. Thus, a signal was given to strangers that this was a person who was bereaved, and was thus liable to emotional volatility and was to be treated carefully and with respect. Quite simply, this does not exist in Britain any more. There are no signs. This is important, since what has been identified here is a tension between feelings and behaviour, a bottleneck, or emotional traffic-jam. It is clear from this that there is some room for stress over and above that which is natural following a death. Thus we see that culture interacts with our feelings in ways which can be detrimental to our health.

According to Parkes (2000) we define **psychosocial transitions** as life changes which have three characteristics. They charge people with revising their world and restructuring it, they are lasting or permanent, and they occur suddenly or over a short period of time. Most of the time, death fits these criteria. Such events often precede the onset of mental illness. That is, it appears that major life events can trigger depression, or other problems. Parkes argues that we make assumptions about the world, and they feed our routines. Someone close to us becomes part of our routines. We ask them for advice, we may share food with them, and a bed, and so on. When we lose them, we may find ourselves rather lost. We still need their advice, their comfort, but they are unable to provide it, and the situation is irreversible. Parkes expresses this as follows:

> Grief following bereavement by death is aggravated if the person lost is the person to whom one would turn in times of trouble. Faced with the biggest trouble she has ever had, the widow repeatedly finds herself turning toward a person who is not there. (p. 327)

Two things must be said about this. Firstly, it is no surprise that mental illness can ensue when a person is placed in such a situation. Secondly, this boils down to an issue of social support, which as health psychologists we know a great deal about. Grief, especially that centred around the death of a life partner, is about the loss of the greatest source of social support.

CONCLUDING REMARKS

As we have seen, chronic illness involves coping mechanisms not unlike those discussed in our chapter on stress. In fact, chronic illness represents a major stressor. In this sense, it is like terminal illness, which is, for many people, the greatest stressor of all. Our reactions to this stressor are determined by many things, including our experiences, our personality, and our culture. The future of palliative care is likely to be one where all of these factors are considered when the dying person is cared for and supported.

This chapter has omitted many of the important and under-researched issues in chronic illness and palliative care, dealing mainly with the basic details. Chronic illness and dying are difficult enough in average adults, but when a person has a learning disability, or is five years old, or both, the issues are possibly completely different. Whilst some exploratory work has been done, more is required. If health psychology is to be inclusive, then such topics need to be researched in order for more and more people to benefit from it.

Study questions

1. How many chronic illnesses can you think of? What are the similarities and differences between them?

2. To what extent is childhood palliative care different from that designed for adults?

FURTHER READING

Kastenbaum, R. (2000): *The Psychology of Death, Third Edition*. London: Free Association Books.

  Probably the only comprehensive book on this topic, and written by someone who has devoted his working life to the study of the psychological understanding of death.

Papadopoulos, L., Bor, R. and Hawk, J. (1999): *Psychological Approaches to Dermatology*. Leicester: British Psychological Society.

  For many, skin disease is a chronic condition. A good introduction to a small but important area of research.

10

Screening

INTRODUCTION

Doctors, and other health professionals, do things to people. People react to the things that doctors and other health professionals do to them. Sometimes those reactions are beneficial to the individual, sometimes they are detrimental. They might be healthier as a result of what is done to them, or they might become unhealthier, especially if their reaction is at odds with the process of cure. This is really a description of a health–behaviour scenario. A main strand of health psychology is the study and development of understanding of people's reactions to things which are done to them.

Screening is one of the most commonly studied procedures. It is the testing of a population to determine which individuals are at risk from, or have developed, a particular disease, impairment, syndrome, or other characteristic. Screening can take the form of a blood, saliva, or urine test, or may involve DNA testing from a scrape of skin from the inside of the cheek. It can also involve a test of one of the senses, such as hearing. Many of us have had our hearing and vision tested at school. Both are screens. One 'golden rule' of screening is that we should only test for things we can do something about. Screening should never be conducted to determine prevalence of a health threat which doctors are unable to ameliorate or eradicate. The argument is that if nothing can be done to help someone, they really ought not to know, especially if the threat is only a potential one or is unlikely to become serious for years or decades. If screening does not increase the health of a nation, it is not appropriate to do it. Most doctors agree that it should never be done solely for the purposes of collecting epidemiological data (statistics on prevalence).

Screens come in two main forms: universal and targeted. A universal screen is applied to everyone in a population, regardless of their individual characteristics. Targeted screens are applied only to people who, research has identified, are in at-risk groups. Obviously, targeted screens tend to be less expensive than universal screens. Both, however, are relatively expensive procedures in medical terms. Imagine that a person's life can be extended by ten years if a particular genetic trait can be identified by screening. Now imagine that only one in 100 000 people actually develop the life-threatening disease associated with the genetic trait. For every million people tested, 100 years of additional life will be gained. However, let us imagine that the total cost of testing one person is £20. So, for a gain of 100 years of life, £20 million must be spent. That works out at £200 000 per year of life. To doctors, this is a lot of money to spend. Very few operations cost this amount, and those that do often elongate life for well over a year. Breast cancer screening, for example, costs a lot of money to conduct. Costs include identifying at-risk individuals, notifying them and inviting them for screening regularly, employing health professionals to carry out the screening, and buying the equipment required. However, this will always be the case for screening. In order to help and save some people, many perfectly healthy people will be tested. In addition, as will be seen, all tests have an associated error-rate. Errors in medical matters can be expensive in a number of ways.

Testing healthy people comes at a cost to the individual, not just in terms of money. Screening raises health issues in people who might otherwise not have been concerned, and one might argue that since they are perfectly healthy they need not have been concerned in the first place. Some people have objections to screening procedures, especially when they are for rarer diseases, particularly because of this. Raising awareness of a health problem can be detrimental to a healthy individual, especially when they are an anxious person. As Marteau (1993) has indicated, some people are made anxious merely by being invited to participate in a screening programme. To certain individuals, being informed by a health professional, either through consultation with their doctor or by post, that some form of investigation is necessary or advisable, implies that something must be awry. People might be suspicious as to why they are being advised to be tested for cancer, for instance. The natural, initial reaction would be to think that the doctor is suggesting this because they believe that you really do have cancer, rather than because you fall into a category of people who are a little more likely to develop certain forms of cancer than other sectors of society.

The screen yields a test result. This is the outcome. There are four possible outcomes of screens. They are called **true positives, true negatives, false**

positives, and **false negatives**. A true positive is when the test shows that the person has a particular disease, and they really do have it. A true negative is when the test shows that the person does not have a disease, and they really do not have it. False positives are when a person is told that they have a disease when they do not. Finally, false negatives are when a person is told that they are healthy when they are not, because the screen has failed to detect the disease. One can easily imagine the reactions to each that a person might have, but health psychologists have studied these in some detail, especially the false results. False results of both categories commonly make dramatic news headlines. The truth of the matter is that all tests have a false result rate, and the sign of a good test is one which has a low false result rate, not one which has none. In developing a screen, doctors aim for a high detection-rate and a low error-rate. Generally, acceptable false positive rates are 5% or below. For instance, Davis *et al* (1997) recommend no higher than a 2–5% false alarm rate for neonatal screening for congenital hearing impairment. We should remember, however, that 5% means that there is a 1 in 20 chance that any given test carried out will be erroneous.

Let us now imagine the potential reactions a person can have to each of the four categories of result, considering research into these reactions where it has been conducted.

TRUE POSITIVES

This is where the person is told that they genuinely have a disease or the potential to develop it and/or pass it on to their children. They may accept or deny the diagnosis, and there are recognised ways and means for dealing with such reactions. The whole force of medical support swings into play when a person is told that they have a 'medical' problem. In a way, a good half of this book is devoted to people who actually have some health problem, as is the majority of medicine. Here we must divide up the reactions into those of people who are told that they have a disease and those who are told that they have a propensity for it.

Knowing that a disease or illness is present can be upsetting for the individual, but they are then able to work with doctors to be cured or to minimise the harmful effects of the problem. Faith in doctors is not harmed, generally, by this, because the person has not experienced any error.

Being told that there is a potential for disease is slightly different because the person is told to take steps to avoid becoming ill and so on, even though they are currently not ill. They might be told that they ought not to have children without prior medical consultation, or that they are likely to become very ill later in life. They might even be told that there is a possibility that they themselves will never become ill, but they have the propensity to do so. Some people may question the doctors' advice, especially those who have no symptoms, and who over time do not seem to be developing any. As time passes, their belief that they are actually at-risk may dwindle, itself a threat to health if certain protective behaviours are dropped. If the screen is for a genetic disorder, research by Henderson and Maguire (1998) suggests that people may be more fatalistic about the outcome. The view is that if something is in the genes it is fixed, immutable and potentially irreversible. Sometimes a true positive result merely confirms what a person already knew. Genetic testing can reveal a propensity for colonic cancer. Reeve *et al* (2000) interviewed seven people who had undergone such testing. In most cases participants suspected, because of family history for instance, that they were prone to cancer. Therefore, in this study, the distress caused by the positive screen result was seemingly at a minimum. We must, therefore, be aware that confirmatory positive test results are much less likely to cause distress than those which are more experimental, where the results may come as a surprise to the individual concerned.

TRUE NEGATIVES

This is an interesting category of people. People with a true negative result are the people that doctors essentially turn away from to direct their attention to the clinically needy. After all, they are the people that we have determined do not require doctors' services. The problem with this approach is that it denies any reactions, thoughts and feelings that a person might have when they have been 'tested' in some way and found to be healthy. Not all people have heard of or thought about a particular health challenge until it is publicised. Health threats can be publicised through the very measures intended to dampen down those threats, namely medical procedures, such as screening. A person might be unaware of the dangers of diabetes until they are tested for it. They start to think about one more health threat. Sometimes the results can take a while to be processed and released. Some people will experience considerable anxiety during the hiatus. The relief of being given the all-clear is enough for some people, but for others the concerns have set in. Some people have a tendency not to believe what doctors tell them. Those people may reject the test result, and start to notice symptoms which they believe are indicative of the disease. They may return to the doctor, asking for further examination and more tests to be done. These are performed at a cost, of course, since no medical system is free. Ultimately, therefore, the psychological characteristics of people interact with the medical procedures designed to reduce challenges to health, perhaps creating new challenges.

Negative results, but particularly true negatives, can encourage an unhealthy lifestyle, in theory at least. As Marteau (1989) suggested, the relief of receiving a negative result, of the all-clear, can actually cause a person to indulge in more health-threatening behaviours. A negative test for HIV, for instance, might make a person more likely to engage in sexual practices which put them at greater risk of contracting the virus. The illusion of invulnerability can be strong when a person has been told that they have escaped a problem which they feared might have affected them.

Another sector of the screened population who receive true negatives may feel that their time has been wasted, and in some cases may resent what they may see as unnecessary infringements upon their lives. The irony is that 'healthy' people are tested for no reason other than to help to identify those people who are not healthy. That is the purpose of a screen after all. Of course, for some screens thousands of people will be tested for every one true positive case. Individuals will have their own opinions on the effectiveness of such a screen, regardless of the true medical value of it.

FALSE POSITIVES

At the time of disclosure of results, one cannot distinguish between a true and a false positive. Again, a proportion of people will challenge the result. Those who do may subsequently have a re-test which yields a negative result. Their confidence in the screening procedure (and in their doctor) might suffer as a consequence. However, most people will accept the result, and then start to come to terms with whatever difficulties they are likely to have to face, now that they 'know' that they have cancer, or carry the gene for cystic fibrosis, for instance. Of course, a tremendous amount of energy might be wasted preparing for something that might never happen. Some false positive test results are never detected. Imagine a test for something where doctors suggest that, if positive, there is a 50% per cent chance that a person will develop symptoms. If a person never does, this is not suspicious, even though the reason why they have not developed symptoms is that they cannot because they are not actually prone to the threat. They might, however, have spent their lives in a state of preparation for something which can never actually happen to them.

A Canadian review of six breast cancer screening trials indicated that as few as 1 in 14 women who are given a positive mammogram result actually have malignant breast neoplasm (Wright and Mueller, 1995). The remainder have benign tumours, or some other non-cancerous condition, or no breast problem at all. Although follow-up procedures tend to detect this, there are still delays of days or even weeks before the patient is told that a mistake has been made. In that time, the patient has undergone undue worry.

Fletcher (1997) reported a common case of misdiagnosis which, although not detected through screening, illustrates the problems associated with false positive diagnoses. An analysis was conducted of saliva samples from 12 000 children which their doctors had stated were suffering from measles. The results were that 97.5% of diagnosed cases of measles were actually something other than measles, leaving the doctors correct in only 2.5% of cases. Although measles is in itself a relatively harmless illness, one of the viruses responsible for spots (which are then mistaken for measles) is the parvovirus, an agent which can cause foetal deformities. Therefore, the false positive, in this case mistaking something for measles, means that some far more dangerous problems may be being left undetected.

Baillie *et al* (2000) report on a qualitative, interview-based study of women's reactions to false positive results of ultrasound screening for chromosomal abnormality. By this method of screening, women can be told if their unborn baby is likely to have certain health problems and disabilities, including neural tube defects such as spina bifida. However, according to the researchers, less than 2% of initial positive tests turn out to be indicative of genuine chromosomal abnormality. This means that 98% of people given a positive result have nothing to be concerned about. Baillie *et al* (2000) interviewed 24 women who had been given a positive screen result but who were subsequently told, after a further round of testing, that the result had been incorrect. A number of themes were drawn out from analysis of the interview transcripts. The ultrasound scan was accepted as a routine part of antenatal care, although a positive result was seen as more serious and indicative than is actually the case (bearing in mind the high false positive rate). There was a perceived shock as a result of the seemingly sudden jump from a routine test to a situation where the women believed that they had a potential termination of the pregnancy to face. For some women, their pregnancy seemed to have become something quite different from the natural process which they had been part of previously. Upon receiving a subsequent all-clear, the women expressed relief, but this gave way to some degree of suspicion surrounding the pregnancy. After all, if the doctors had been mistaken about the result once, they could be mistaken again, perhaps. In at least one case, this created doubts about having children in the future. What this shows is that the process of screening carries with it various possibilities for those who undergo screening, and that there is not a single fixed feeling associated with the routine, but a series of emotions and cognitions which may last beyond the pregnancy itself. Whilst, for some, screening represents a good way to enable mothers to understand their pregnancy and make choices, for others it can be a stressful process. The authors suggest that women need to be better prepared for the results of a screen.

FALSE NEGATIVES

The greatest problem that a false negative result generates is an illusory sense of well-being. People are told that nothing is wrong, but really something is wrong. At the point of the giving of the result, there is no difference between a false negative result and a true negative one, since neither doctor nor patient knows that the false negative is false. Again, some people will challenge the result, and in this case to good effect since a further test may yield an accurate result. Others, intuitively one would say the majority, will accept the result, and assume that all is well. Of course, in time they may start to develop the disease screened for, and their presenting symptoms may be such that a doctor orders a second test. Should this prove positive, some patients will be angry at the doctor, and some will have their confidence in the whole testing or screening procedure, and possibly the medical profession itself, taken away. This can have important consequences for their subsequent treatment, since their adherence may be significantly affected.

Some people will have some concerns about symptoms prior to being tested/screened. So, a false negative result can be alarming, since they are convinced that something is wrong, but are being told that their conviction is unfounded.

DANGERS OF SCREENING AND TESTING

Like virtually all medical procedures, when screening protocols are carried out there is a level of risk associated with them. Antenatal screening for Down's syndrome using amniocentesis (the drawing off of a sample of the fluid from around the foetus in the sac) can cause miscarriage for instance in around 0.9% of cases (Wald *et al*, 1997). Parents are thus often faced with the dilemma of accepting this risk in order to know if their child is likely to be affected or taking no risk but not having the information.

Swedish neonatal testing for α_1-antitrypsin deficiency was abandoned after two years because doctors (rather than their patients) expressed concerns about parental reactions to the screening process (Thelin *et al*, 1985). Here is a clear case where additional problems can be created by a procedure put into place to enhance, rather than threaten, health.

Mammography screening (to detect breast cancer) involves using radiation to 'view' the tissue contained within the breast. Of course, radiation is harmful to us, and there are still arguments between biophysicists and others about what levels are considered 'safe'. Ironically, the best method for detecting breast cancer involves subjecting the breast to x-ray radiation. Radiation causes cancer. Although the doses of radiation involved in mammography are small, there is a risk, however negligible. Whilst the occasional additional cancer might be created when hundreds of thousands of women are screened, a figure acceptable to doctors compared with the number of women whose lives are saved, it is difficult to imagine a woman feeling happy to sacrifice her own health for the sake of that of others. Additionally, mammography also involves high pressure on the breast to flatten it out in order to achieve the best radiographic image at the lowest doses of radiation. However, some doctors believe that manipulating tumours can increase their rate of metastasis (spreading to other areas). So, if a tumour is present the process of screening can exacerbate the situation, however slightly. For women who are aware of these issues, they may represent significant obstacles in the path of adherence to screening.

Once a test is completed and the result available, the way in which the outcome is communicated to the patient can have a great impact on how it is understood and acted upon. A note of caution is necessary concerning the terms used by doctors in describing test results. Tluczek *et al* (1991; 1992) point out that the average person might misinterpret the words 'positive' and 'negative' when they are used for test outcomes. Most of the time, 'positive' equates with 'good' and 'negative' with 'bad'. People say things like 'try to be positive' and 'don't be so negative'. Of course, when it comes to tests for diseases, genes and the like, the connotations are reversed. Negative is an all-clear, and positive rings alarm bells. If health professionals do not make this clear, some at-risk or affected individuals might believe that they are safe.

In the box below is a genuine letter from a general practitioner to a patient, with only the personal details and dates changed to protect identities.

Dr. S.G. Kenwood-Heath
The Lawns
Ternford
Tel: 033 987654321

14th May 2000

Dear Ms Crompton

We have received the result of your Cervical Smear test taken on 10/4/00. The result of your test was negative, therefore no further action is required.

Yours sincerely,

S Kenwood-Heath

S.G. Kenwood-Heath

If a person believed that a negative test result was bad, the sentence containing this word could be seen as a highly alarming statement. The doctor's statement that no further action was required could be interpreted as a comment that the person has an incurable cancer and that there is nothing that medical science can do for them. To some people, this letter might be interpreted as information to the effect that they are going to die and that there is nothing more that can be done. Not only might this cause considerable upset, but it is also likely to cause further costs of time and money, since the confused recipient must contact the doctor again for clarification, thus taking up the doctor's time. A clear and thorough letter sent initially would avoid both the unnecessary upset and the secondary contact.

Compare this with the fictitious letter (below) which explains, in simple terms, the outcome of the test, avoiding any ambiguities.

Dr P.G. Lenton-Carvey
6, Tenfield Grove
Carmonston
Tel: 099 1234567

Dear Ms England

We have received the result of your Cervical Smear test taken on 6th October 1999. The result of the test was negative. This means that you have no abnormalities and therefore your cervix is healthy. No further medical action is needed. Your next routine test should be in two years' time and we will contact you again nearer that time to arrange an appointment. Should you have any questions about this test, or your health in general, please contact the Practice Nurse, Mrs Patricia Goss, on the above telephone number.

Yours sincerely,

PG Lenton-Carvey

Dr P.G. Lenton-Carvey

However, it is not only patients who are open to confusion and misunderstanding. Sadler (1997) has pointed out that even health professionals (in this case general practitioners, obstetricians and midwives) can be lacking in knowledge about screening and testing procedures. In this study of Down's syndrome serum screening testing, large proportions of health professionals incorrectly answered questions about it, general practitioners being the least informed of all groups compared. As a result, information-giving to patients is often done poorly. Marteau *et al* (1992) looked at antenatal information-giving about screening and found that different health professionals gave varying information to patients and that spending more time with the women did not mean that more information was conveyed.

Some studies have identified bias in patients' memories of screening results. This means it is important that when results are given they are given clearly and unequivocally. With respect to cholesterol testing, people enrolled in Croyle *et al*'s (1997) study showed a memory for their cholesterol rating which was often inaccurate, tending to misremember in the direction of safety rather than danger. People remembered being healthier than they actually were, in essence. The longer the time between testing and recall of result, the greater the discrepancy between the real and the recalled result. The more the true result was in the unhealthy direction, the greater the mismatch between memory and the true cholesterol score. Over time, it seems, people have a tendency to forget information related to their health, reconstructing the memories in a way that best suits the preferred state of affairs: good health.

NON-ADHERENCE

This chapter has focused so far on those people who have been screened or tested. Some people refuse, for whatever reason, to take part and be tested. They represent a very different challenge for health professionals and one on which much attention has been focused. Whilst they have the right to opt out of a programme, doctors would prefer it if all people who should be screened or tested actually were. French *et al* (1982) looked for the reasons for non-attendance at a breast-screening clinic. Their research aimed to identify if non-attendance was mainly due to individual characteristics such as personal experiences or personality, or due to characteristics of the service being provided (such as accessibility, staff competence and so on). They discovered that fear of finding out that they had cancer put women off attending. Non-attenders were more likely than attenders to see the breast clinic as a place where bad things happen, rather than a place where good occurs. Of those who attended, a small proportion felt that a diagnosis of cancer would seriously alter their lives, whereas almost three-quarters of non-attenders did. Therefore, ironically perhaps, fear of cancer and its ramifications can prevent people from attending screening to ascertain whether or not they have cancer. The irony lies in the fact that the screening process is used to identify those people in danger in order to deal with that danger as effectively as possible. By non-adherence, those women who did not attend the breast screening clinic increased the possibility that they would actually die from breast cancer. This demonstrates that health beliefs and health values are often based not upon 'logic' but upon more emotive factors.

Certain demographic factors seem to affect whether people take up or refuse screening when offered to them. Looking again at breast screening, younger, married, middle-class women tend to be more likely to attend screening than older women, single women, or those who are working-class (Vernon *et al*, 1990). It is likely that there are numerous reasons for this. Rather than the reasons being cultural *per se*, it is possible that they are related to other factors, such as health beliefs, which, of course, tend to vary, for instance with social class.

One practical barrier to attendance is the accessibility of the clinic. People from lower socio-economic strata are less likely to have private transport, more likely to be unable to afford child care for the period of attendance at the clinic, and less likely to be able to afford the cost of a screen in countries where healthcare is not funded out of general taxation (Rimer, 1992). It is rare for a person to find that the nearest and most convenient hospital to them provides the full range of services they are likely to need, especially since hospital authorities (in Britain at least) often tend to specialise and to avoid providing services which they feel less able to handle expertly.

Some studies have pointed to doctor recommendation as a factor in screening uptake. Essentially, when people are told by their doctor directly that they are best served by attending a clinic for screening, they are more likely to attend (Aiken *et al*, 1994). However, as Swinker *et al* (1993) have shown, with respect to mammography once more, a good tenth or so of women most susceptible (those over 50) simply refuse screening when it is offered to them by their doctor. Doctors' recommendations to patients to take part in screening must be carefully made. The author knows of one doctor (there will no doubt be others) who sends out letters to women inviting them to cervical smear screening. These letters give a specific date and time when an appointment has already been set up for the woman concerned. They also state, quite correctly, that the woman should be in the middle of her menstrual cycle when the test is performed. Of course, this makes the setting up of the appointment a nonsense, since there is no reason to suppose that the date given will be a mid-cycle one! Women who receive such letters may well question the doctor's understanding of the relevant issues, which can do nothing for their confidence in their doctor.

Another study has demonstrated that peer pressure is also important in determining whether or not women will comply with mammography (Champion and Miller, 1996), showing that people listen to friends' medical advice, not just that of those qualified to give it. If peer influence is important in encouraging women to attend screening, it is also likely to work negatively. Women's bad experiences of screening may be off-putting to their friends. If a women tells her friends that her cervical smear test was painful and embarrassing (which, with a less skillful health professional it can be), her friends might avoid their own screening when it is due.

As you would imagine, perceived susceptibility can make a significant impact on uptake of screening. If a person does not feel vulnerable or at risk, they are much less likely to attend screening than someone who knows or feels that they are likely to be in some danger (McCaul et al, 1996; McCaul, Schroeder and Reid, 1996).

The more the public perceive a test or procedure as dangerous, the higher the amount of non-compliance. Logically, doctors would not create tests which put people at more risk than the risk that the test itself is designed to remove by detecting a problem early. However, people do not weigh up the costs and benefits in this way, but use a much more idiosyncratic, and often illogical, scheme. As we have seen elsewhere, this is why health psychologists create belief and cognition models. If a person believes or feels that a screen or test is 'too' dangerous, they will fail to accept it. However, as Orbell and Sheeran (1993) have shown with respect to cervical smear screening, accurate knowledge of the screen and its benefits is associated with higher incidence of uptake.

Cameron (1997) reports an extensive study of cancer screening in America which is using a health–psychology theoretical framework. The researchers are using the self-regulatory model (see Chapter 3 on Perceptions, Beliefs and Cognitions for details on the model) to consider if vulnerability beliefs, barriers to action, social influence and other factors are contributory to screening adherence and non-adherence with respect to mammography in thousands of women. The researchers found a relationship between belief in personal vulnerability (susceptibility) to breast cancer and a family history of the disease, although the strength of the correlation between these factors ($r = 0.40$) was smaller than one might have logically expected. One would imagine, perhaps, that most people who had a family history of breast cancer would feel particularly vulnerable, resulting in a correlation coefficient of closer to twice this size. This goes to show that, as stated earlier, logical and intuitive expectations are not always borne out by data, because human beings do not follow the rules of logic or common sense. Furthermore, vulnerability beliefs were not found to significantly predict intentions to engage in mammogram screening, but they did affect intentions via a less direct route involving social influence (friends and family may have perceived the vulnerability in the individual and applied pressure to them to attend screening). The author reports that less than 40% of variance in intentions to have a breast cancer screen were predicted by a combination of personal habit (such as whether a person has attended in the past), social influence (such as suggestions by friends that the screen is important to attend) and barriers (such as lack of time or money). Whilst this constitutes some success as far as models of behaviour go, we must not forget that this means that over 60% of a person's screening-intentional behaviour is not explained by the factors the researchers have been looking for. Essentially, we do not know the majority of what is going on. Again, this is not indicative of a failing of health psychology, but of the tremendous complexity of human behaviour. Even the most simple ideas and behaviours are often underpinned by an array of other behaviours, contexts and influences, many of which we have only just begun to investigate through research. As Crossley (2000) states

> If we look carefully at how people conduct and talk about their health-related activities, it becomes apparent that their 'decisions' to act in certain ways do not conform to rational, logical, value-free ways of thinking, but have their own alternative logic and validity that is related in a complex fashion to the cultural and moral environment in which they live. (pp. 38–9)

There is one further reason for non-adherence which should be mentioned, and that is political opposition. In the case of a number of disabilities, some politically motivated people find screening offensive and an affront to their lifestyle and culture. Inherent in the screening ethos is a view that the world is a better place without disease and disability. When people can be screened for certain health challenges and disabilities, many people will choose to avoid having children who will be at risk, either through the choice to avoid pregnancy, or through termination. Those who choose to have a child who is affected by cystic fibrosis or fragile X syndrome or Down's syndrome, for instance, may face discriminatory attitudes. As the population of people with certain disorders diminishes because of preventative technologies, so fewer resources will be available for that dwindling minority of people who require them, and negative attitudes may occur such as the view that people who choose to have a child when they know that it will be disabled are 'irresponsible' and 'a drain on the system'. The argument is that eradication of disability is a desirable and achievable state of affairs. However, to say that the world would be a better place without, for instance, people with Down's syndrome in it, is highly distasteful to a great many people. It is seen as no more acceptable than suggesting that the world would be better without black people in it, or women. This kind of 'disablism' is understandably seen as no less than a form of health-Fascism. Health promotors are often accused of health-Fascism because their work is to try to persuade others that certain forms of living are superior to others because they are healthier. Naturally, those people who object fundamentally to these kinds of approaches will be much less likely to take part in screening programmes than those who do not.

There is evidence that negative attitudes can be formed towards those people who refuse screening and are perceived, therefore, as snubbing doctors' efforts to create a healthier world. Marteau and Riordan (1992) asked health professionals to rate their feelings about fictitious patients who had or had not attended a screening programme for cervical cancer and had subsequently developed the disease. The participants showed more negative attitudes towards those who had not been screened than those who had, suggesting that even amongst health professionals there is a tendency to have less sympathy, perhaps, for those people who developed a disease after failing to avail themselves of a preventative measure offered to them. This, of course, might have ramifications for the treatment those individuals receive from the doctors and nurses. Gerbert (1984) demonstrated that doctors gave more information to patients that they liked than those that they disliked, even though all presented with the same symptoms. There is already some evidence for the institutionalisation of this kind of thinking in British hospitals, with smokers being prioritised lower than non-smokers for treatment of certain smoking-related diseases.

CONCLUDING REMARKS

We have seen in this chapter the multitude of reactions which people can have to screening procedures. The perceptions and emotions differ from person to person, and can be affected by a range of factors, including the information provided about the screening procedure and the manner of the people responsible for it. One difficulty presents itself to researchers in this area. As health psychologists learn more about human reactions to medical technologies, the technologies develop further, in some way invalidating the previous work. As every new type of screening procedure appears, there is more work for health psychologists in understanding people's feelings about it. Whilst it means that there might be no shortage of research for us to do, it also means that in a constantly changing field it is difficult to establish a body of knowledge which is stable.

Study questions

1. Is fear of the consequences of non-vaccination a good way to encourage people to be vaccinated against diseases?

2. Imagine that a vaccine existed that could prevent the development of all forms of heart disease completely. However, there is a ten percent chance that it will kill a person who takes it within five years. Would you take it? Why?

FURTHER READING

Lee, L., Brittingham, A., Tourangeau, R., Willis, G., Ching, P., Jobe, J. and Block, S. (1999): Are reporting errors due to encoding limitations or retrieval failure? Surveys of child vaccination as a case study. *Applied Cognitive Psychology*, 13, 43–63.
  Parents often cannot remember if their child has had their vaccinations. This study suggests that rather than simply forgetting, parents did not really take the information in in the first place.
Marteau, T.M. (1989): Psychological costs of screening. *British Medical Journal*, **291**, 97.
  A somewhat dated but nevertheless groundbreaking paper outlining the effects that screening procedures have on people.

11

Mind and Body, Placebo and Pain

- Introduction
- Placebo effects
- Tastes, colours and shapes
- The experience of pain
- Concluding remarks
- Study questions
- Further reading

INTRODUCTION

The mind and body are not separate things, at least in terms of their functioning. If there is one thing that this book is intended to teach you, it is this. Throughout the book there are many examples of the relationship between thoughts, feelings and actions and the way that the body works. Two of the clearest ways in which it can be demonstrated that the mind and the body work closely together are with respect to placebos and the experience of pain. A placebo is a neutral substance which can have a curative effect on a patient, even though pharmacologically it ought not to. It is not a 'real' drug, or a 'real' therapy. Of course, for the people for whom it works, it is very real, and very effective. Pain affects virtually all of us, bar those rare individuals for whom the nervous system has developed abnormally leading to a total absence of pain sensation. Most days, most of us experience some pain, however slight. We might even have occasionally done something to 'take our mind off the pain'. It works, to some degree, when we do. We even speak of mental pain, although the sensation of mental pain, is, of course, a different one from bodily pain. Here we examine the ways in which health psychologists, amongst others, have studied both placebo effects and pain.

PLACEBO EFFECTS

Most doctors will accept that all of medicine is associated with some degree of placebo effect. No matter what is done to treat a person, part of the strength, or effectiveness, of the treatment will be due to a placebo effect. This applies to both orthodox medicine and complementary approaches, such as Chinese medicine, ayurvedic medicine, reflexology, homeopathy, and so on. Placebo literally means 'I will please', and there is much to be gained from appreciating this; being pleased is a psychological phenomenon.

Hawthorne and placebo effects

Firstly, we ought to distinguish between a true placebo effect and a Hawthorne effect (Roethlisberger and Dickson, 1939). The Hawthorne effect is where change itself acts as a solution to a problem. It was first discovered in an industrial setting, but it is also relevant here. Changes to levels of lighting in a factory altered levels of dissatisfaction amongst workers, regardless of what the change was. The workers were made temporarily happy by seeing that the employers were doing 'something' to improve conditions. When a patient is given a new drug, some of the placebo effect will actually be a Hawthorne effect; anything different works for a while because the patient is getting the attention of the doctor. It may even explain why some doctors try patients on a series of drugs, each only working for a few weeks or months.

The true placebo effect, as Ernst and Resch (1995) point out, is what is left after comparing the real drug's effects with the placebo effects, balanced against a no-treatment group. Very few studies ever include a genuine untreated group, often for ethical reasons. However, this means that the size of the placebo effect is, possibly, seemingly greater than it really is. Sometimes groups of people show improvements without any treatment whatsoever. Spontaneous recovery is, in milder conditions, quite common. After all, the body is constructed in such a way as to fight illness; that is what the immune system is for, for example. People often tend to seek medical help at the point where their illness is at or nearing its peak, because they leave it for a while in the hope that it will cure itself. At the point where a person is recruited into a study, they may be on the road to self-recovery. Therefore, what appears like a placebo effect may actually not be. What Ernst and Resch (1995) argue is that studies into the placebo effect should have three groups: drug, placebo, and untreated. If a painkiller removes 75% of pain, and a placebo removes 25%, the untreated group tells us what the true placebo effect is. If an untreated group shows reductions in perceived pain of 10%, then the placebo effect is only 15%.

Researching placebos

Naturally, placebo studies need to be randomised, and double-blind. A randomised study is where people are assigned to the experimental (real drug) group or the placebo group entirely randomly. From a list of patients, for instance, assignment to groups can be done alternately. The first to experimental, the second to placebo, and so on. A double-blind study is one where the patient does not know whether they are in the experimental or placebo group, and nor does their doctor. The co-ordination of the study is achieved from a central point from which the doctor is sent the drugs they must give to the patient. The doctor does not know if they are giving a real or a sham drug. This is very important, since, even subconsciously, a doctor may treat patients differently if he or she knows which group they are in, thus ruining the study. One further note: we have been speaking of drugs here, but placebo effects apply to all therapies and interventions, including psychological ones like counselling, and surgery. Studies of surgical techniques often have mock surgery groups included. Patients are left with a scar from a wound, but they are not aware that nothing has been done to them. Many people are uncomfortable about the ethical issues surrounding such work. When patients are recruited into a double-blind study, they are told exactly what their chances of receiving a placebo will be. However, once in the study they do not know if they are receiving the real therapy or the placebo. The false hope that this might create is a source of ethical debate.

How placebos might work

We can now look at some of the findings of placebo research, and what they tell us about the relationship between mind and body. For placebos to work, it is likely that certain conditions have to be met. The variable factors are the attitude/motivation of the patient, the attitude/motivation of the doctor, the characteristics of the treatment, and the nature of the illness. Research has tended to focus on one or some of these, but few studies try to model placebo success based upon all of them.

We can envisage a number of scenarios based upon combinations of the above. Imagine a patient with a mild illness, who has faith in their doctor. The doctor believes that giving them a placebo will be helpful, and communicates this belief in the 'treatment' to the patient. The treatment is convincing enough, since it involves taking a combination of yellow and red pills at various times of day. There are even side effects, since the doctor has given what is known as an **active placebo**, which mimics the effects of a real drug but does not have the therapeutic advantage. In this circumstance, the chance of witnessing an improvement in the patient's condition due to the placebo is high. However, let us now consider the opposite. We have a patient with a life-threatening illness who has little confidence in their doctor, and is quite opposed to taking medicines. The doctor shows poor faith in the medicine they are prescribing, since they describe it as 'quite experimental' and just say that 'it's worth a try'. It comes in the form of a capsule which reminds the patient of a jelly bean. Not surprisingly, placebo effects in this case are much less likely to appear. Of course, health psychology is more interested in subtle effects, rather than such obvious extremes.

There is research to show that the attitude of the doctor or therapist is important, and that any sign to the patient that the doctor is not confident that the therapy will work is likely to reduce the patient's faith in the treatment too. As a result, not only might a placebo fail to work, but an active drug might also lose some of its therapeutic effect. As early as 1956, Feldman showed that a genuine tranquilliser lost 67% of its effectiveness when a doctor presented it to a patient as something which he had doubts about. It became almost useless when the doctor took away its credibility. In fact, the effectiveness of a drug which can be due to placebo effects is quite often greater than the effectiveness of a real drug after faith in it has been lost by a patient.

The attitude of the patient is also implicated in the placebo effect. Having faith in something can make a big difference to how it is perceived and interpreted. Movies are often 'hyped' for a good reason; the money would not be spent otherwise. By building up to a film and making it seem amazing, people feel that it must be true, and when they see it they perceive it as a better movie as a result. Of course, some people will reject the publicity and the opposite will occur, but for many publicity is a positive force which makes them view things as better than they might otherwise. Similarly, a person who believes that the laying of crystals on the body can promote healing is likely to report some change in their symptoms as a result of a session of crystal healing. This may occur partly because they interpret any changes in the illness as being due to the crystals, but also because their belief may trigger additional work by the body's own healing systems. This latter point is something which is still to be extensively researched. So, patient attitude and motivation are key factors in the generation of a placebo effect. Jensen and Karoly (1991) separated out expectation from motivation. The former is a patient's *belief* that a treatment will effect a cure or cause a change in illness state, and the latter is the patient's *desire* to be cured or perceive a change in symptoms. They gave people a mock sedative, and found that although both factors predicted the size of the placebo effect induced, motivation contributed more. This means that if we wish to make use of placebo effects we must work with a patient's need to get better rather than trying to convince them that a treatment can be effective.

Further to the issue of patient motivation and expectation there is that of **demand characteristics**. This term is used by psychologists to describe the thoughts and feelings of a person who takes part in a study *about* the study itself, but is also applicable to the thoughts and feelings about the clinical consultation by a patient. Essentially, people try to figure out psychological experiments, and their behaviour, either consciously or unconsciously, begins to match what they think we are likely to be investigating. They almost 'want to please' the researchers, by 'doing the right thing'. Of course, this is all supposition, since they don't really know what the researchers are investigating

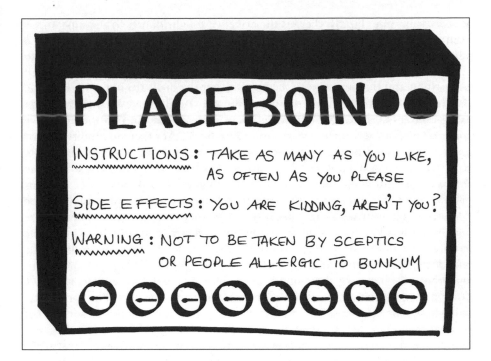

quite a lot of the time. Occasionally, some people will try to ruin a study by behaving in opposition to the perceived purpose, but most people have a more philanthropic attitude, and try to behave in a way which they see as appropriate. Similarly, when doctors give patients a prescription, many patients do not want to let the doctor down by failing to get better. These strong social psychological forces can be responsible, in some part, for observed placebo effects. This can work in two ways. Firstly, individuals may report a reduction of disease symptoms where there isn't really one. This is not always something the doctor can verify. Therefore, some people might tell the doctor that their pain has gone, thanks to the 'treatment', when in fact they are still in pain. They feel that they cannot tell the truth, because to do so would be to tell the doctor that he or she has failed, somehow. Of course, the doctor usually has to take the patient's word in a case like this; pain is an area where we have to rely on self-report. Secondly, patients may themselves experience a reduction in symptoms because their desire to please the doctor is so strong that they alter their perceptions of their illness to suit the treatment being applied. They stop noticing their pain as much, they concentrate on episodes without pain, and so on.

There are a number of other mechanisms through which the placebo effect might work. Some or all of these explanations may be true in any given patient at any given time. Firstly, there is the effect of conditioning. When a person is used to something happening, a special cause–effect bond is created. When a person smokes a cigarette, they feel some positive things, and they learn to associate those things with smoking a cigarette, thus making the bond difficult to break. Placebo effects might be a learned response to a stimulus. In this case, the stimulus is a drug or a therapy of some sort. People have learned to expect some relief of symptoms from being given a treatment, and so they perceive some relief even when the treatment is not 'real'. Another possibility is that anxiety is lowered by the treatment, even when it is a placebo. In the case of pain, for instance, if a doctor tells a patient that they are being given something that will alleviate their pain, they feel relieved and less anxious. Now, anxious people tend to feel more pain than people who are relaxed, and so pain will be perceived as less strong simply because of a reduction in general anxiety. Since perception is a key factor, we must mention attention. Although it is possible to perceive without attending, most of the time we tend to perceive more of the world that we attend to than the world we ignore. When we attend to something, it takes on greater significance. This is obvious. Of course, when we don't attend to something, it fades out of our consciousness. Placebo effects may show themselves because a patient is told that they will notice some relief of symptoms. This focuses their attention on the periods of time when the pain, or itching, or whatever, undergoes some remission. Even without treatment, illnesses ebb and flow. If we take eczema as an example, people who have this skin condition will report periods of time when it is particularly bad and periods when it has almost disappeared, regardless of any treatment. If a person is primed to focus on the latter, they will associate the treatment with the remission of symptoms, even when the treatment is fake (Ross and Olson, 1981). They may distort time, so that the condition-free periods are perceived as longer and the flare-ups as shorter than they actually are. Thus the natural progress of a disease over time is combined with a distorted perception to create a strong placebo effect.

The placebo effect also might work through the stress–health relationship. Receiving a real or perceived treatment might, in itself, lower anxiety and stress in an individual. As we have seen elsewhere, stress is associated with ill-health, and better recovery is often a product of a reduction in stress levels. Placebos can be particularly effective when the illness has no discernible organic origin, that is where the doctor cannot find anything physically wrong with a patient. In such cases, since the illness may be largely psychological, so is the cure.

Cognitive dissonance is a concept which we have met with before in this book. To remind ourselves, it is essentially Festinger's (1957) idea that when we make choices in life we often do so in such a way as to reduce dilemmas and tensions that arise. The theory of cognitive dissonance has been applied by health psychologists in attempting to explain the placebo effect, although this alone cannot explain all of the phenomenon. In essence, a placebo does nothing to us in any medical sense. When we take a placebo, nothing happens. Of course, we have been given a 'treatment' by the doctor, and so we expect it to work. We invest a lot in modern medicine. We pay for it, either directly through private systems, or indirectly through our taxes, or in a combination of the two such as is in operation in Britain. (The National Health Service is paid for mainly from general taxation, but most working people must pay for prescriptions and dental work.) We also invest time and effort in going to see the doctor, and we believe that what the doctor does for us will help us. So, when we are given a drug which has no effect, cognitive dissonance occurs. We need to avoid feeling cheated, or stupid, or misled, and we must uphold our investment. We have a choice, however subconscious, of rejecting the doctor and turning our back on our investment, or of creating a situation where the drug actually does work for us. The placebo effect is just this. We choose to 'trick' ourselves into believing that the drug really has worked, and by focusing our attention on the positive, and ignoring the negative, we have a good result.

Totman (1987) gives a good account of this experience of cognitive dissonance and how it can lead to placebo effects. According to Totman, people usually like to justify their behaviours, both to themselves and to others, and they must also feel like they have control over what they do. (We have seen in other chapters how important a sense of personal control, with respect to health is to people.) When a person invests in a treatment which does not seem to work, the dissonance occurs because the person chose to seek and accept this treatment (control), but the act of doing this cannot be justified because it did not work. A reframing of the situation so that the treatment is perceived to work reduces the dissonance, and all is well. Totman argues that this explains the placebo effects which allegedly underpin a great many complementary medicines. Non-standard health interventions are big business, and if people did not perceive them to work, at least to some extent some of the time, then they would simply give up on them. We know that many people have a great deal of faith in their favourite complementary therapy, just as many people have strong religious faith. Of course, applying the cognitive dissonance argument to religion would be an insult to millions. Those people who invest in complementary medicines might be equally annoyed at Totman's suggestion that they do not work other than by convincing the person that they had better find use in them since they have paid a lot for them. One problem with this theory is that it relies upon non-conscious mechanisms which are left unspecified.

Placebo effects are not always found, even when the circumstances for their fostering are ideal. Merikle and Skanes (1992) investigated possible placebo effects associated with subliminal self-help tapes. Subliminal self-help audiotapes rely upon a hypnosis-like effect, whereby people are given suggestions to eat less, stop smoking and so on, below the level of conscious hearing. Very, very quietly, there is a voice on the tape, making suggestions to the listener.

They cannot 'hear' them consciously, but there is some evidence that people can still take in information that they are not consciously aware of. Have you ever walked down the street and thought about someone only to see them immediately afterwards? This usually happens because you *have* already seen them, but the fact of having seen them has not entered conscious awareness. You think of the person, but you don't know *why* you do. Merikle and Skanes (1992) examined the placebo effect in overweight women who firmly believed that such tapes could help them to lose weight. Thus the right conditions for an observed placebo effect were ensured. The participants were divided into a 'real' subliminal tape group, a mock subliminal tape group, and a control group who were given no tape at all. The women in the real and mock groups were not aware of which type of tape they had been given. Over the course of the study, all three groups lost weight, and the average weight loss was the same for all groups. Thus, placebos cannot be assumed to be present for all remedies and cannot be assumed for the most 'gullible' or faithful people. Furthermore, the study provides some evidence to suggest that such methods of weight loss are not actually worth pursuing for most people.

TASTES, COLOURS AND SHAPES

There is even research to show that the form of administration of a drug, and its colour, alters its effectiveness. You may have wondered why pills come in a variety of shapes, sizes and colours. It is not just for aesthetic reasons. In the scheme of things, making a drug look pretty is not really important. However, most chemicals in pills are not naturally brightly coloured. Most are white powders of some sort. Colourings are added. The first reason is a practical one. If all pills looked identical, then a person taking four or five pills a day could mix them up, with disastrous consequences. Another reason is that there is a strong placebo effect associated with colour, and drug designers can use this to their advantage. If a drug is 60% effective in its natural form, but 75% effective when a red dye is added, then the manufacturers would be foolish not to take this into account. That 15% is the placebo effect.

Medicine is rarely pleasant. To stop children finding pills and munching on them like sweets, they are often given a bitter taste, just as natural gas, which is normally odourless, is given a smell by the gas suppliers so that you notice when there is a leak. Furthermore, pills which taste 'like medicine', that is they are unpleasant, are likely to be associated with a stronger placebo effect than those which do not. The placebo effect relies upon authenticity, and we characterise authentic medicines as tasting bad and looking slightly sinister at times. Pills are something that you really shouldn't touch unless you need them for an illness. Thus, a placebo which mimics these aspects of real treatments is more likely to work (Shapiro, 1964). 'Good' treatments are specific, rather than vague. When the doctor tells you to take 'a few' pills 'now and then', the message being sent out is that the pills are harmless. After all, if they could harm you, the instruction would be far more strict and specific. Of course, if the pills are harmless, they can't be that great for curing your problem. In these circumstances, placebo effects are likely to be operating at a minimum, if at all. When the doctor tells you to take one a day, with lunch, avoiding dairy produce, and to tell her if you experience any headaches or rashes, the drug sounds dangerous. For dangerous, read effective. The placebo effect is maximised in this scenario.

De Craen *et al* (1996) report a systematic review of the 12 existing studies into the colour of a drug and its influence on perceived effectiveness. A systematic review is a special type of research where all of the research on a particular subject is summarised and synthesised. If there are consistent findings across all research, then those findings take on greater credibility. What De Craen *et al* (1996) found was that red, yellow and orange drugs are generally perceived as stimulating, whereas blue and green ones are often seen as tranquillising. One study compared blue and orange sleeping pills. People who took blue capsules fell asleep more quickly than those taking orange ones, and they also slept for longer. In another study of patients with rheumatoid arthritis, patients were given either real painkillers or placebos coloured red, green, blue or yellow. Whilst the real painkillers were equally effective regardless of colour, there were differences amongst the placebos. Blue and green placebos did reduce pain, but the red placebo was as effective a painkiller as the real drugs. What this suggests, of course, is that there is an argument here for saving money on painkillers and administering red placebo pills, at least in some circumstances. Without resorting to conspiracy theory, one must remember that people generally have no inkling that they have been given a placebo. This means that we all could have been given placebos in the past without ever knowing. Of course, with such a profound psychological influence on pain relief, 'psychological pills' (placebos) can be a legitimate part of the treatment process. Such a dramatic description of the psychological nature of the treatment of pain is probably a good starting point for a discussion of pain and the perception of it.

Before that, however, it is helpful to summarise the factors involved in the placebo effect. Placebo effects may occur because of a combination of the following.

- **Patient expectations:** if the patient believes in the treatment, and wants to get better, then the conditions are right for placebo effects.
- **Doctor expectations:** if the doctor has a belief in the treatment, this encourages placebo effects.
- **Conditioning effects:** through people's lives they associate doctors with getting better. Therefore seeing the doctor provokes feelings of health.

- **Stress and anxiety reduction:** being 'treated', even falsely, reduces anxiety and stress, thus engendering the conditions for health.
- **Misattributions and altered perceptions:** naturally occurring changes in the illness are mistakenly attributed to the effects of the 'treatment'. People focus their attention on certain signs and away from others, which gives the impression of a cure being effected.
- **Degree of credibility of therapy:** greater placebo effects are associated with treatments which are perceived as *bona fide*.
- **Demand characteristics:** people want to please the doctor, and so get better, or report getting better, in order to do so.

THE EXPERIENCE OF PAIN

Pain is a word we all use, and a feeling most people understand. However, if you take two people and ask them to describe a pain which you have controlled so that the sensation should be as similar as it is possible to make it, they will give you different accounts of it. There will be similarities, but there will be differences. They may agree or disagree on whether or not it is a stabbing pain, or an ache, or whether it is a hot or a cold pain, or on how long it persists. This is the fascinating aspect of pain, and also what makes it so difficult to study properly. Study it we must, however, because pain is a significant factor in the decisions which health professionals have to make about the quality of life of a person. If you only have the resources to treat one person today, you might want to choose the one who is in the most pain. Of course, how do we know? Is the person who wails the most the one experiencing most pain? Not necessarily: it all depends upon the person. The first published acknowledgment that pain has a strong psychological component comes from Beecher (1946; 1956) who looked at requests for pain relief (analgesia) amongst soldiers and compared these to the requests made by civilians with the same injuries. Most of the soldiers claimed not to perceive any pain and only a quarter of them requested pain relief. In the case of civilians, over 80% asked for analgesic support. He argued that the context in which the pain was experienced had an impact on the way in which it was perceived.

Pain is not even something that all human beings avoid all of the time. Have you ever felt pain that was enjoyable? Sometimes we prod a bruise to encourage the pain, and provided that the pain is mild it can be a pleasant sensation. During sex, people may engage in grasping and biting which causes, again, mild to moderate pain. Some people are interested in sexual pain beyond this 'normal' level, and are masochistic. Certainly, it seems, the psychological component of pain can override the physical one.

Theories of pain perception

Early pain theories focused on the physical or physiological aspects, trying to understand what was happening at the level of tissue damage. This approach, dominated as it was by reductionism and a strong medical-model stance, was doomed from its onset, simply because it has always been known that pain has a substantial psychological component. What then happened was a growing interest in the psychological aspect of pain. However, there was a clear mind–body dualism about this. Pain which was caused by physical factors was termed **somatogenic** or **organic pain**, and that which was 'in the heads' of the perceivers was termed **psychogenic**. Of course, the problem with this view is that it separates out what might be called 'real' pain and that which is 'imagined'. A perceived pain, according to this approach, is *either* psychogenic *or* somatogenic. Most pains are likely to be both at once. If you stub your toe against a door, the body has suffered an obvious injury. Thus, one expects pain. The pain is clearly somatogenic. However, some people can stub their toe and just say 'ouch', whereas others will need to sit down for ten minutes, rubbing the toe, and will continue to experience pangs from it for hours to come. Furthermore, a person who normally tolerates pain quite well will, on occasion, be more susceptible to it, for instance when they are very busy or very stressed. A person who is normally pain-intolerant may become quite tolerant when they are excited and happy. There is clearly a mixture of psychological and physical components to every pain, and that is why theories developed on from this basic state of affairs. Hope and Forshaw (1999) demonstrated that with respect to low back pain, which commonly appears to have no somatogenic origin, physiotherapy is not always effective, and that the effectiveness of it is related to the amount of psychological distress that patients are experiencing.

The most enduring and famous theory of pain perception is the **gate-control theory**, espoused by Melzack and Wall (1965). According to gate-control theory, there is a barrier at the level of the spinal cord, which acts as a gateway for incoming and outgoing signals associated with the sensation of pain. When the gate is fully open, pain is perceived at its strongest, and when the gate is closed there is no pain. Of course, most pain signals are being transmitted via a partially open/closed gate. The gate is opened and closed by a combination of physical, emotional and behavioural factors. Almost all pains are made up of psychological and somatic components, although at different times one may predominate over the other.

The gate can be opened by physical factors such as bodily injury, emotional factors such as state of mind, anxiety and depression, or behavioural factors, such as attending to an injury and concentrating on the pain. Similarly it is closed by physical factors such as analgesic remedies, emotional factors such as being in a 'good' mood, and behavioural factors such as concentrating on things other than the injury.

According to Melzack and Wall (1982), there are three dimensions which contribute to our experience of pain. These are *sensory–discriminative*, *affective–motivational* and *cognitive–evaluative*. The first of these refers to information about the location of a pain, its intensity, and its pattern over time. The affective–motivational dimension concerns our motivation to act on the pain, and the cognitive–evaluative facet is where our experiences of past pain may shape our perception of current pain. In combination, these dimensions of pain shape the overall pain experience.

Sensations have different effects upon the gate, and different sensations compete with each other to get through the gate. Why do you rub yourself when you have pain? It is, seemingly, an instinctive thing to do. Well, rubbing is friction, and some people have suggested that friction signals compete with pain signals to pass through the gate. In fact, they appear to compete successfully. If both signals are trying to get through, the friction signal will make it first. Continuous rubbing will mean that the pain signal has little chance to be 'heard' in the nervous system. This may also explain part of the phenomenon that pain sensations are reduced during sexual intercourse. This involves friction, of course, and of highly enervated (supplied with nerves) parts of the body. Pain signals, therefore, may fail to get through the gate. Since gate-control theory also allows for psychological components, the context of a sexual encounter will also close the gate somewhat.

Gate-control theory would, theoretically, suggest that there is a limit to the physical pain that can be experienced. After all, an open gate cannot be 'more' open. Of course, this cannot be tested empirically, but the fact that some people in intense pain lose consciousness might suggest that the gate has been opened fully, and losing consciousness could be a protective mechanism to prevent some kind of 'overload' to the system. This is by no means an accepted explanation, however. The hyperventilation that some people undergo when in excruciating pain could account for this.

This theory also, implicitly, calls into question laboratory-based, experimental research on pain. If perceived pain is influenced heavily by mood and by environment, then the work done on pain in laboratories is unlikely to give us much information about real-world pain experiences. This lack of **ecological validity** is a serious problem with experimental pain research in general.

Whilst gate-control theory is a serious step forward in accepting the various contributory factors in pain perception, a problem with the theory is that it is difficult to quantify the effects of the individual factors. Just as pain itself is difficult to assess and attach a value to, so we run up against difficulties when we try to work out which factors are more important than others, and so on. Imagine that we wanted to 'calculate' perceived pain in an individual, using the suggested factors from gate-control theory. A person has a sudden-onset headache. Let us say that the gate is 60% open/40% closed. (We have to begin with an assumption, since there is little way of evaluating even this.) When the person takes some aspirin, how much will the gate close? If the person is in an anxious mood and has recently seen a TV programme about brain tumours, how much will this open the gate? We simply have no way of making these calculations, which means that the theory has a very limited predictive value. In psychology, we tend to favour models and theories which allow us to make predictions.

Gender and pain

There is some evidence to show that men and women differ in their reactions to pain. Using methods such as cold-pressor stimulation (see below), women show lower tolerances of pain than men. However, women can tolerate considerable pain in certain circumstances, such as during a difficult childbirth or in dysmenorrhoea. Women typically report more pain than men, and are more likely to report pain which is difficult for doctors to ascribe to a particular cause. Of course, there is no way of separating out the social norms operating from genuine differences in biological functioning. Men, in most of the societies where psychological research is conducted, are expected to be 'tough' and to accept pain. As a result, men may feel pain but are less likely to report it to a doctor.

Women present a good example of another phenomenon of individual difference research; that of variation in baseline performance. People not only differ from each other in various measures, but also differ from themselves at various points in time. There is evidence that women's tolerance of pain fluctuates with the menstrual cycle. In the middle of the cycle, women tend to be more sensitive to pain (Gijsbers and Niven, 1993). However, women who experience painful menstruation do not tend to show this variation in pain-sensitivity. In fact, they show levels of tolerance to pain lower than average throughout the month. The suggestion is that the hormone prostaglandin is responsible for both the dysmenorrhoea and the pain sensitivity.

One important way in which this information on sex differences can be useful is when a doctor is making a judgement as to which patient of two ought to be treated first, based upon self-report of pain, all other things being equal. If one were male and the other female, an understanding of the average differences in pain tolerance between men and women may assist in the decision, as may some knowledge of the menstrual status of the woman. Again, when comparing two women in pain, menstrual status could, theoretically, be built into the decision-model. For any particular woman who is regularly visiting her doctor because she is in pain which is being monitored, it is essential that the doctor is aware of the cycle of the woman so that comparisons of pain experienced from week to week take this into account.

It is very important, however, not to reduce women's experiences down to explanations involving gender, hormones and the menstrual cycle, since there are a great many other factors influencing pain-sensitivity. Such knowledge must be handled tactfully and in a way that does not imply or promote sexism.

Phantom pain

Phantom pain is the term used to describe pain which quite simply, on the face of it, should not be there. People who have had limbs removed often report pain sensations in the limbs. They feel a pain where their hand should be, for instance, even though there is no hand. The pain is, essentially, in thin air.

Two other types of unexplained pain are worth mentioning here (Melzack and Wall, 1982). *Neuralgia* is pain that occurs along a nerve and is intense and shooting in nature. The face is often affected. The pain is so strong that it often distracts the person from doing anything. There appears to be no reason for the pain, no tissue damage or the like, but folk myth often explains the pain away by exposure to cold, such as the wind. *Causalgia* is a burning pain which is felt at the point at which a previous wound existed. Whilst only a small number of patients who have been wounded experience causalgia, for those who do it can be debilitating. Both causalgia and neuralgia can be triggered by external stimuli, which can be of the mildest nature (such as a kiss or a slight breeze).

Possibly the most important point to consider in pain of this nature is the reaction that the individual may have to it. Support may be required in the form of advice from a health professional. A person feeling things in an arm which does not exist may be quite frightened, and may even doubt their sensations. Without support, they may believe that they are experiencing hallucinations, and are, therefore, 'going mad'. Pain without reason, such as neuralgia, can be distressing for a person. As cognate beings, we seek explanations for things. We assume that pain is there for a reason, and that the reason is that something is wrong. Without anything obvious to point to, people can become anxious and think the worst. Of course, by this point in the book you will know that the next point to be made is that anxiety can lead to stress, and that stress causes or exacerbates ill health. Thus a cycle is established, pain causing stress causing pain causing stress. For these reasons, 'meaningless' pain needs to be explained to a patient.

Measuring pain

If we wish to study and understand people's idiosyncratic perceptions of pain, we have to be able to measure it. A commonly-employed and very basic measurement of pain can be achieved through the use of what is called a visual analogue scale (VAS). Here people are asked to rate the intensity of their pain by making a mark along a line which represents a scale from 'no pain' to 'unbearable pain', or something similar. By measuring the distance along the line the person has made the mark, we can get an index of how much pain they are feeling. A problem with a VAS is that only the intensity of pain can be recorded in this way, not the quality of it, that is whether it is burning or piercing or throbbing. It is also not a method of measurement which works well when trying to compare different individuals to discern who is experiencing the greater pain. Quite simply, there is no way of equating the pain experiences of two people. It is no different from the difficulty of assuming that two people 'see' the same thing when they see the colour blue. They can both recognise blue, but it does not mean that they actually see the same thing. The best use for a VAS is when comparing an individual's pain with their pain at another point in time. Since we can expect some steadiness in responding based upon a person's character or general resting level of behaviour, we can assume that mostly a rise or fall in reported pain on a VAS does relate to a true rise or fall in perceived pain. Since using VAS instruments does not give information as to the *type* of pain being experienced, more sophisticated tools are usually needed.

Possibly the most well-used pain-perception measurement tool is the McGill Pain Questionnaire (MPQ) (Melzack, 1975). The MPQ is an instrument which recognises that there are a number of dimensions to pain, in terms of its quality. Pain is not just about intensity, but about type. Thus we have hot and cold pains, dull and sharp pains, and so on. Earlier we noted that the gate-control theory suggests that pain consists of three dimensions: sensory–discriminative, affective–motivational and cognitive–evaluative. These three are reflected in the construction of the MPQ. People are asked to rate the intensity of the pain (a quantitative index), along with the type of pain experienced (a qualitative index). A person is asked to choose from a list the words which best describe their pain, and then give a rating of the intensity of that feeling by numbering each word selected. For example, a person can choose between 'sickening' and 'suffocating' to describe their pain (but may not choose both), or may deselect both terms. Of course, those people who would like to describe their pain as both sickening and suffocating in equal amounts will not be well served by the MPQ.

Another problem with the MPQ is that it is not always possible for a patient to liken their pain to one of the descriptions given. Given that there is such a wide variation of perceptions, some patients would prefer to use their own words to accurately describe what they are experiencing. Sometimes patients simply do not know what some of the words mean. Do you know what 'lancinating' means? If you are fortunate enough that you do, ask a few people around you. You will find that a large majority do not. This word appears in the MPQ. Similarly, not all people use words in exactly the same way. How can we be sure that a 'smarting' pain to one person is the same as a smarting pain to another. What smarts to one person may sting to another. Furthermore, the words 'taut' and 'tight' appear in separate categories in the MPQ. To many people, these words may seem synonymous. Of course, this is not to say that

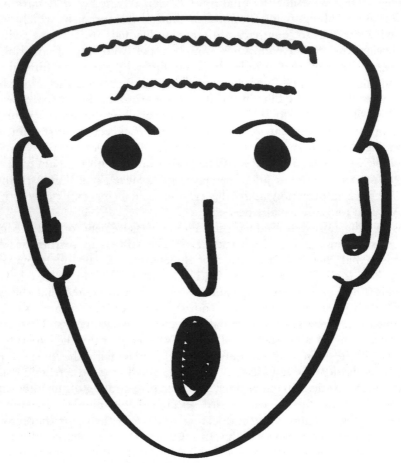

WELL... IT'S A KIND OF ACHING,
STINGING, STABBING, BURNING
THROB THAT GNAWS AND BITES
... SORT OF... ITCHY... AND...
EXCRUTIATINGLY MILD...

the MPQ is not an excellent questionnaire. Quite simply, given the nature of the phenomenon, all other instruments to measure pain are likely to be equally flawed, if not more so. Measuring the idiosyncratic or personal is always a problem for psychology, and the fact that we will never do it perfectly is not a reason for giving up.

Whilst self-report is probably the best way to assess pain, it is not the only one, and occasionally some extrinsic measure of pain, based upon a person's behaviour, is used. This is especially valuable when faced with patients who are likely to lie about their pain, either neurotically or strategically exaggerating it to gain attention or some other benefit, or making light of it either because of denial, or not wanting to bother others. In these cases, there can be a discrepancy between self-report measures and a behavioural index. The most commonly used method in experimental pain studies is **cold-pressor stimulation**. It is a measure of tolerance to pain. You will probably know that if you put your hand into cold water for a while, pain results. Cold-pressor stimulation is a controlled version of this. A person places their forearm in room-temperature water for a minute, then in a special apparatus in water at 2°C. They must hold down a platform, under the water, until they can no longer stand the pain. At this point, reducing pressure on the platform will allow it to spring back upwards, taking the arm out of the water. The value of such a method is that people are being asked to tolerate the pain for as long as possible, and the experimenter can be sure that pain is actually being experienced. However, the social–psychological issues still pertain. Just because a person has said that they cannot tolerate the pain any more does not mean that they have genuinely reached their threshold of tolerance; they may have reasons why they would like to appear more intolerant than they really are. This is something which may affect the studies of pain and gender across many cultures. Whilst women seem to be less tolerant of pain in general than are men (Goolkasian, 1985), this might be an effect exacerbated by a social pressure on women to appear 'weaker' and more 'dainty' or 'ladylike' than men. Where such social pressures exist, women may be less likely to push themselves to tolerate pain. The converse applies to men, of course, in such cultures.

Managing pain

A serious issue for health psychologists is in working out ways in which people can manage their pain, especially people with chronic pain. There are many medical methods for dealing with pain, such as surgery and drug treatments, but equally important are psychological interventions aimed at enhancing a person's ability to cope with pain. These are especially important in those situations where the pain is not well managed by traditional doctors' methods.

Distraction is one psychological method. Earlier we discussed the role of attention in the placebo effect. By shifting attention away from pain, people can actually feel less of it. Some dentists attach teddy bears to their clinical lamp, so that children will notice that and ignore the treatment. Have you noticed that some people swear and shout when they hurt themselves? Again, this could be nature's way of introducing a distraction. However, distraction may not always work. Whilst it is good for weaker pains, intense pain is not always best dealt with by distraction. Sometimes pain is so strong that a person needs to concentrate or focus on it in order to manage it. If you have ever experienced intense pain, you will probably know what it means to be unable to think of anything other than it.

Pain redefinition involves giving the pain experienced a new meaning. In many ways, pain redefinition is a cognitive–behavioural-therapy approach. Thoughts about the pain which are negative are replaced by more constructive and positive ones. People may be taught to think that the pain is not as bad as it is, or they are taught to have faith in their ability to cope with the pain. In one sense, the first of these is a form of denial, which as we have seen elsewhere, can be a good strategy for certain people with some illnesses some of the time. Saying to yourself 'it's not really that painful' when it is actually very painful is a lie, but people can believe their own lies. If the lies can be therapeutic, then it makes sense to take advantage of them. Let us now consider an example of pain redefinition, within a loose cognitive–behavioural framework.

Case in Point: Lucy

According to psychologists, people have, in their minds, schemes for how the world works, how things happen, why things happen, and so on. Such a set of beliefs is called, rather transparently, a **schema** (plural, schemata).

Lucy developed low back pain three years ago, and has experienced episodes of it on at least a weekly basis since. She is referred to a psychologist, who assesses her and believes that her pain can be reduced by redefinition. She clearly has some negative thoughts about the pain which need to be addressed. People often have 'internal sentences' which they repeat to themselves, in various paraphrased forms. Lucy's internal sentences, the psychologist believes, are adding to her pain.

The psychologist has identified some of these as follows. Upon feeling pain, Lucy thinks to herself:

- This isn't right . . . this means something is really wrong with me . . .
- Oh no . . . it's happening again . . . it's never going to stop.

- What am I going to be like in a few years?
- This is going to get worse and worse.
- I will be permanently disabled if this carries on.
- This is really frightening . . .

According to her doctors, Lucy's condition is stable, and so most of her fears are unfounded. Therefore, it is quite appropriate for the psychologist to work with her to remove these debilitating ideas. Once the ideas are identified, substitute sentences are created, in negotiation, which will have a calming effect on Lucy. At first, it may help to have these written on postcards, to be referred to when she starts to feel overly negative about her pain. On cards, she may have new sentences like:

- The doctor says that my condition is stable.
- I can trust the doctor. She is very experienced.
- I can cope with the pain I have now. It won't get worse.
- The pain is a sign for me to be careful. I can look after myself and keep this in check.

By redefining the pain, and by introducing a coping element into Lucy's cognitions, slowly Lucy can be encouraged to develop a new schema for her low back pain, which doesn't involve fear, which does involve positive coping strategies, and which turns the pain into a useful signal for Lucy to engage in health behaviours which will protect her against further injury and pain. Eventually, the postcards should not be needed. The aim is to permanently replace her negative thoughts, so that dealing with the pain is entirely in her mind.

Such an approach depends strongly upon words. Words can, at times, seem trivial, but to a person they can be the most important thing. An experimental study by Koutantji, Pearce and Oakley (2000) looked at the processing of pain-related words in people who experienced either a high amount of pain, or a low amount. They concluded that people who experience a lot of pain develop biases towards processing pain-related words. This can have an effect on their world view: '. . . one's frequent pain experience could create a self-schema of the 'self in pain' where selective-processing of pain-related material occurs. This might also have implications for processing of other self-relevant information and the general organisation and content of self-knowledge' (Koutantji, Pearce and Oakley (2000), pp. 285–6).

Imagery techniques to reduce pain essentially involve thinking about something else to take the mind off pain. Pleasant scenes like holidays and birthdays and wholesome meals are imagined, and the pain weakens as a result. Of course, not all people have visual imagery that is strong enough to support this technique (and some have none at all). For those who have, it can be effective. It makes sense to view this as a form of distraction, at least in some ways. By thinking of something else, people are distracted from the pain.

Hypnosis is another technique, relying upon psychological phenomena, commonly used to treat pain. A number of dental surgeons now use hypnosis as an alternative to anaesthesia, with considerable success.

However, hypnosis does not work for everyone. Hypnotherapists tell us that there is no point trying to hypnotise a person who does not have faith in the phenomenon of the hypnotic state, or who does not want to be hypnotised. Here we come around full circle, since the same rules govern placebos to some extent. Those who are most susceptible are likely to benefit most (Barber, 1982). Without belief, they often do not work. The difference is, of course, that in the case of placebos the faith is in the 'real' treatment which patients may believe they are receiving, whereas, in the case of hypnosis, faith must be placed in the hypnotic procedure. There is no such thing as a placebo for hypnosis. The hypnotic state is defined, for most therapists, by the patient themselves. If they think and feel that they are hypnotised, then they are. There is no objective, external verification of this state of consciousness. Hypnosis, then, represents a wholly psychological therapy with distinct uses in medical settings and in enabling individuals to control their own health. In the dental arena, hypnosis has two main uses. It can be applied in cases of worried patients, to reduce their anxiety. Anxiety can actually reduce the effectiveness of surgical anaesthetics. It can also be used as an alternative to anaesthesia, for patients who are allergic to it or have some other objection. Since, in Britain at least, general anaesthetic has been ruled out in most dentists' practices because of the danger to life associated with it, hypnosis is beginning to present a feasible alternative for some patients.

CONCLUDING REMARKS

Throughout this chapter we have seen examples of the relationship between the mind and the body, and there is little doubt that much of what goes on in the body also goes on in the mind. There are many other areas where mind and body interact strongly, and the rest of the book has dealt with some of them. Health psychology itself is all about mind and body. Even the reductionists, those people who claim that all phenomena can be reduced to a common denominator such as atoms or quanta of energy or neurotransmitters, end up admitting that mind and body are linked, since they would argue that the mind is actually a product of the body. Damage the brain, and you damage the mind. It is a little more surprising to suggest that the mind affects the body, but if we take many of the examples from this book, there are some simple demonstrations of it. Self-harm is one of them. A state of mind causes a person to alter their body, physically. Of course, this is a long way from arguments about mind-over-matter. This is something which health psychology can offer some evidence for, but there is not necessarily anything supernatural about this. Psychoneuroimmunologists are just beginning to explore the mechanisms by which what goes on in the head influences what goes on in the body. Whilst we spend energy seeking mechanisms behind phenomena, we must be aware of one thing which affects all human endeavour after truth. Essentially, the more we learn, the more we generate questions, and the more we realise we still need to learn. Human beings are probably the most complicated things we could ever choose to study, and as a result, psychologists have a difficult job to do. Cultures change over time, and people change over time, which means that studying people is like trying to draw a moving object. But our methods of observation and experiment also change over time. It is probably better to say that studying human behaviour is like trying to draw a moving object with a pen that keeps turning into a pencil, then a brush, then back to a pen again. It is a challenge which anyone who steps into the world of academic or practical psychology undertakes.

Study questions

1. Clap your hands together, or pinch the skin on your hand or leg. Write down what it feels like, how long the sensation lasts, and whether the feeling changes over time. Get a friend to do the same, then compare your descriptions.

2. If you were inventing a placebo, what would it look like and why? What would you have to consider in creating it?

FURTHER READING

Kuhn, M.A. (1999): *Complementary Therapies for Health Care Providers.* Philadelphia: Lippincott Williams and Wilkins.
> Everything you ever wanted to know about complementary therapies, along with summaries of the research for and against them. The best starting point if you want to work out which therapies are mainly placebo and which are not.

Horn, S. and Munafò, M. (1997): *Pain: Theory, Research and Intervention*. Buckingham: Open University Press.
   An excellent short book on the whole topic of pain. Part of a series of books covering a range of health psychology topics.

Glossary

This glossary is meant as a quick guide to some of the terms used in this book. It does not provide fool-proof and exact definitions of the terms, since in most cases exact definitions are almost impossible to give in a few words.

ACTIVE PLACEBO

A placebo which mimics the effects of a therapeutic drug, i.e. has side effects without the therapeutic effects.

ADHERENCE

A term used to denote how a patient 'sticks to' medical advice. This term is, today, used instead of 'compliance'.

ANALGESIA

Pain relief, which can be effected physically, using chemicals, or psychologically, using cognitive techniques or hypnosis.

ANOREXIA NERVOSA

A mental illness where a person starves themselves in order to be thinner, mistakenly perceiving themselves to be fat no matter what their size.

APPRAISAL SUPPORT

When a stressed person is encouraged or enabled to evaluate their own state of health and are thus able to put their stressors into context, appraisal support is the name given to this.

AVERSION THERAPY

A therapeutic process whereby people are 'put off' doing things by associating them with unpleasant sensations or thoughts. To stop someone eating chocolate, aversion therapy might involve giving people chocolate flavoured with a bitter substance.

BEHAVIOURISM

A school of psychology which concentrates on explaining human behaviour in terms of conditioning. Behaviourists believe that all non-instinctive human behaviour is a product of learned associations between stimulus and response.

BINGE EATING DISORDER

This is similar to bulimia nervosa (BN), but without compensatory activity. That is, instead of eating large quantities and then purge–vomiting as is typical of BN, people with binge eating disorder simply tend to eat the large quantities *per se*.

BIOFEEDBACK

A form of therapeutic process through which people can learn to alter their physiological processes by watching them change on some kind of meter. For instance, relaxation can be taught by showing a person the physiological indicators of relaxation and training them to control their bodily responses to create a relaxed state.

BIOPSYCHOSOCIAL MODEL

The prevailing model of health within health psychology. The focus is on the interaction of the mind and the body and there is an acceptance of the range of individual differences in personality and culture which can affect health. More consideration is given to how the life of an individual is affected by their illness and vice versa.

BUFFERING HYPOTHESIS/DIRECT HYPOTHESIS

These are hypotheses about how social support brings about reductions in stress. In the direct hypothesis, social support is directly good for you, whereas in the buffering hypothesis social support acts as a buffer, cushioning the individual against major stressors but having little impact on minor hassles.

BULIMIA NERVOSA

An eating disorder. People tend to eat large quantities of food (and sometimes non-foodstuffs such as linen) and then vomit or take laxatives to prevent the intake of calories having an impact on their weight.

BURNOUT

A term used to describe the syndrome affecting people who have experienced stress and fatigue in their work over a long period of time. It is characterised by lack of empathy for others, loss of perceived self-efficacy, and exhaustion.

CALIBRATION

The accuracy with which people can judge their own knowledge about something.

CENTRAL NERVOUS SYSTEM

Essentially, the brain and spinal cord.

CHRONIC ILLNESS

Any illness which is likely to last a long time or a lifetime. It is contrasted with acute illness.

CIRCADIAN RHYTHMS

Biological rhythms or cycles which can create patterns of behaviour. Our sleep cycle is an example. Disturbances of these rhythms can create serious health problems, and health problems can cause disturbances of the rhythms.

COGNITIVE DISSONANCE

A feeling experienced when there is some degree of contradiction between two outcomes. When a person does something for themselves which also harms them in some way, cognitive dissonance is felt. For example, if a person spends a lot of money on a holiday, they might harm themselves by creating financial difficulties. In order to reduce cognitive dissonance, they must believe that it was 'worth it', that they have benefited from the holiday and that it has been good for their health.

COMPLEMENTARY/ALTERNATIVE MEDICINE

Health practices and systems like reflexology and homeopathy which purport to heal using mechanisms other than those used by orthodox medicine. Doctors prefer the term 'complementary' medicine, since 'alternative' implies that orthodox medicine is not required at all.

COMPLIANCE/NON-COMPLIANCE

The extent to which a person adheres to medical advice and/or a treatment regimen. The term is now ill-favoured, and 'adherence' is mainly used instead.

CONDITIONING

This refers to the pairing up of actions and their reactions. Pavlov first demonstrated this by showing that if a dog learned to associate the ringing of a bell with food, the bell alone would produce salivation after a number of such pairings.

CONFRONTING

This is a coping strategy which involves dealing with a problem by facing it and by arguing out problems with people.

CONTENT VALIDITY

In psychometric evaluation, content validity refers to the extent to which the content of a test is appropriate for the tool to be able to assess what its makers purport that it assesses.

CONTINGENCY CONTRACTING

A form of reward system used in therapies such as cognitive–behavioural therapy. The client enters into a contract with the therapist which means that certain things will be given or withdrawn depending upon the client's behaviour.

COPING

A significant term in health psychology, it is used in a range of contexts, none of which are at odds with the normal dictionary definition of coping.

CRONBACH'S ALPHA

A method of analysis of responses to questions which form a scale. Cronbach's alpha gives an index of the relationship between responses to questions which are meant to be asking similar things. The higher the alpha value, the greater the internal reliability.

DEMAND CHARACTERISTICS

The perceived demand upon an individual taking part in a study. What a person perceives as the purpose of a study can affect how they behave or answer questions that they are asked.

DENIAL

A refusal to accept that a health problem exists. A common coping strategy.

DEPERSONALISATION

Viewing others as if they are not thinking, feeling people but rather as objects or as units of production. This is a characteristic of 'burnout'.

DISPOSITIONAL OPTIMISM

A built-in optimistic view that can have ramifications for health, either positively, by adding to 'fighting spirit', or negatively, through 'denial'.

DISTANCING

A form of coping with a problem or stressor in which a person distances the problem from themselves, perhaps by laughing about it.

DOUBLE-BLIND PROCEDURES

Used mainly when testing out drugs, an experimental method whereby neither doctor nor patient knows if the drug being given is active or a placebo.

EMOTIONAL SUPPORT

A form of social support which, as it sounds, refers to being loved, cared for, and listened to.

EMOTION-FOCUSED COPING

Contrasted with problem-focused coping, this involves addressing and working through one's emotional reaction to a problem rather than dealing with solving the problem itself.

ENDOCRINE SYSTEM

The hormone-producing glands of the body which are responsible for regulating many of the body's mechanisms such as thirst.

ESCAPE AVOIDANCE

Coping with a problem by avoiding it. This is classic escapism such as 'drinking to forget' or 'throwing oneself into one's work'.

ESTEEM SUPPORT

Social support which takes the form of others showing an individual that they are valued and respected.

EUSTRESS

Positive stress, which may be good for the individual. Some people appear to thrive on moderately stressful situations. In addition, the exhilaration felt from watching a horror movie or riding a rollercoaster is very similar to the feelings during acute stress, although the context is all-important in determining the way that the situation is perceived.

EXTERNAL RELIABILITY

The extent to which a test gives us the same scores from individuals upon re-test. This is only a good measure of the strength of a test when we actually expect the scores to stay the same upon re-test. It is especially important when re-testing relatively stable factors.

FACE VALIDITY

The extent to which a test or other instrument appears, on the face of it, to be assessing what it is intended to assess.

FALSE NEGATIVE

A test result which tells the patient that they do not have a disease or illness when they actually do.

FALSE POSITIVE

A test result which tells the patient that they do have a disease or illness when they actually do not.

FIGHTING SPIRIT

A term used to describe a personality characteristic which some evidence suggests might enable a person to defeat certain illnesses.

FIGHT-OR-FLIGHT RESPONSE

A physiological response to an environmental threat. When in danger, the body becomes biologically prepared to either stand and fight or to run away.

GALVANIC SKIN RESPONSE

A physiological measure of stress which involves assessing the degree of electrical conductance of the surface of the skin, which increases in stressed individuals due to increased levels of salts.

GATE-CONTROL THEORY

A theory of pain perception which takes into account the many physical and psychological dimensions of pain and likens the movement of pain signals to the brain to objects passing through a gate of adjustable size.

HARDINESS

A personality characteristic which may predispose people to being more resilient to disease and illness.

HASSLES SCALE

A stress-measurement scale intended to detect stresses caused by minor hassles as opposed to major life problems.

HEALTH ACTION PROCESS APPROACH

A multifactorial model of health behaviours taking into account motivation, self-efficacy and personal will.

HEALTH BELIEF MODEL (HBM)

A model which helps to predict health behaviours based upon perceptions of susceptibility to an illness, costs and benefits of the health behaviour, and environmental 'cues to action' which can trigger the behaviour.

HEALTH BELIEFS

A term used to denote the thoughts and folk knowledge that a person may have about health. For example, a person may believe that one glass of brandy a day promotes health.

HEALTH VALUE

The concept of the value people place upon their health in general or particular health behaviours.

HOMEOPATHY

A complementary therapy involving the consumption of 'tinctures' of plant extracts, which are heavily diluted with water, often to the point where no molecules of the original substance are present in the therapy. Homeopathic therapists argue that the substance leaves a molecular impression on the water molecules, which can have a therapeutic effect.

HOSTILITY

A characteristic associated with Type A personality behaviour.

HYPOCHONDRIASIS

An unhealthy, sometimes disabling, preoccupation with ill-health, where a person believes themselves to be suffering from one or a number of illnesses or diseases when there is no medical evidence that they are.

ILLNESS COGNITIONS

A term used to denote the thoughts and folk knowledge that a person may have about illness. For example, the beliefs that cancer can be contagious, or that the mind can cure the body, are illness cognitions.

IMMUNOCOMPETENCE

General health and efficiency of the immune system.

INFORMATIONAL SUPPORT

Support provided by information, such as books, leaflets, the internet, or knowledgeable individuals and experts.

INSTRUMENTAL SUPPORT

Practical support, such as financial backing or gifts of material goods.

INTELLECTUALISATION

A coping mechanism in illness, whereby people distance their illness from themselves by studying it and speaking of it as an academic, rather than personal, phenomenon.

INTERNAL RELIABILITY

The extent to which questions in a scale are asking the same thing of the respondents.

LIKERT-TYPE SCALING

A type of scale using which a person can respond to a question. Unlike in the 'visual analogue scale', people respond to a statement by choosing one of a set of categories, such as 'Totally Disagree', 'Disagree Somewhat', 'Neither Agree Nor Disagree' and so on.

LIMBIC SYSTEM

Part of the forebrain responsible for certain basic behaviours such as eating, drinking, aggression, anxiety and sexual activity.

LOCUS OF CONTROL

A term used to describe the way in which people ascribe the things which happen to them as being either their own doing (internal locus of control) or the doings of others (external). External locus of control is divided into powerful others and chance (fate).

MEDICAL MODEL

An outmoded view of the human condition which was persistent in medicine for most of its history and is still present in some spheres today. Essentially, the human being is seen as almost entirely reducible to tissues and physiological processes, and the culture, thoughts and beliefs of a person are generally ignored.

MEDICALISATION

A term used mainly by sociologists to describe how the medical profession may have 'taken over' certain aspects of normal life, such as childbirth.

META-ANALYSIS

A form of analysis of the results of experiments which involves adding together various results from similar studies as if they were all part of one bigger study.

OBESITY

Being overweight, commonly defined technically as having a body mass index of greater than 25. This is computed as weight in kilograms divided by height in metres.

ORGANIC PAIN

Pain which has an obvious physical cause.

PALLIATIVE CARE

The branch of medicine devoted to supporting people who are deemed terminally ill.

PERIPHERAL NERVOUS SYSTEM

All aspects of the nervous system excluding the central nervous system.

PHANTOM PAIN

Pain which is perceived in a part of the body which has physically been removed.

PLACEBO

A substance which is inert but which is given to a patient who believes that it has therapeutic properties.

PLANFUL PROBLEM-SOLVING

A strategy for coping which involves planning a way out of a problem state.

POSITIVE REAPPRAISAL

Turning a problem into something positive by looking for ways in which a stressor has benefited the individual.

POSITIVISM

A view, attached to reductionism and the medical model, that there are indisputable 'facts' which are 'out there' for us to discover.

PROBLEM-FOCUSED COPING

Contrasted with emotion-focused coping, this involves dealing with a problem by working through it and seeking practical solutions.

PROTECTION–MOTIVATION THEORY

A development of the Health Belief Model which incorporates a prediction of intentions as a precursor to behaviour.

PSYCHOGENIC ILLNESS

Illness which has no obvious physical cause.

PSYCHONEUROIMMUNOLOGY

The study of the mind and its interaction with the immune system.

PSYCHOSOMATIC ILLNESS

Illness which may have a physical cause but which also has a psychological component.

RANDOMISED CONTROLLED TRIAL

A method of experimentation in medicine whereby one group is given the drug or treatment in question and another group is not. Allocation to these groups is entirely random.

RAPID SMOKING

A way of getting people to stop smoking by asking them to smoke continuously until they are nauseous.

READABILITY FORMULAE

Methods of assessing how difficult a passage of text might be to read.

REDUCTIONISM

The view that all phenomena can be 'reduced' to a common denominator such as sub-atomic particles, cells, chemicals, or physical process. It is a component of the medical model of health and illness.

RESTRAINED/UNRESTRAINED EATING

In the study of eating disorders, terms used to describe people who are either attempting to control their food intake (restrained) or those who eat whatever they like, whenever they like (unrestrained).

RUMINATION

Ruminators are people who, when faced with stress, tend to ponder their problem without directing their thoughts at a solution.

SCREENING

Testing a population or sub-population for a disease, illness or genetic propensity.

SEASONAL AFFECTIVE DISORDER (SAD)

An illness which has depression as its principal symptom and which is a reaction to levels of natural, environmental light.

SELF-REGULATORY MODEL

A model of illness cognitions which attempts to explain adjustments which a person makes to becoming ill.

SET-POINT THEORY

A view that people have a biological set weight which, despite diets and the like, the body works hard to maintain.

SOCIAL COMPARISON

A method of coping which involves comparing one's own health state with that of others, either in the immediate peer group or in the world in general.

SOCIAL MODEL

A view of psychological and social life which holds that many of the realities of our existence are socially constructed, i.e. made up by human beings. One of the most developed areas is the social model of disability, in which it is maintained that in a world where disability is not perceived as important and which is constructed to meet all needs, not just of those who are non-disabled, disability would cease to exist.

SOCIAL READJUSTMENT RATING SCALE

An early scale to measure stress which gives rankings of major life stressors ordered against each other.

STOIC ACCEPTANCE

A term used in the study of coping, especially with terminal illness and grief. Stoic acceptance is a resolution to accept what will be.

STRESS INOCULATION TRAINING

A stress-reduction technique which involves people recognising their own reactions to stress and dealing with them as a result.

STRESSOR

Anything which causes stress.

TARGETED SCREENING

Testing for an illness or a genetic propensity by aiming the tests only at those people who are believed to be at high risk. For instance, babies might be tested for hearing impairment only if a parent is deaf.

TASKS/TESTS

A task is anything which a psychologist asks a person to perform. A test has a more precise meaning, and is a measure of performance, usually intended to allow the psychologist to compare the person's performance with that of others.

TENSION-REDUCTION HYPOTHESIS

A view that alcoholism, and other addictions, arise because the addictive substance has a stress-reducing value for the individual.

TEST BATTERY

A group of tests intended to give a set of scores which help to label, categorise and understand an individual's abilities and/or character.

THEORY OF PLANNED BEHAVIOUR (TPB)

A model of health behaviour, developed from social psychological theory, which incorporates perceived control into the prediction of behaviour, along with subjective norms and attitudes.

TRUE NEGATIVE

A true test result which tells the patient that they do not have a disease or illness.

TRUE POSITIVE

A true test result which tells the patient that they do have a disease or illness.

TYPE A PERSONALITY

A personality type associated with high levels of impatience, competitiveness and hostility. Such people are more prone to heart disease than those with a type B personality.

TYPE B PERSONALITY

Defined principally by an absence of type A personality characteristics.

TYPE C PERSONALITY

A personality type associated with developing cancer. Type C individuals are likely to fail to express anger openly or to 'bottle things up'.

TYPE I DIABETES

Also known as insulin-dependent diabetes. Rarer than type II. Injections of insulin are necessary.

TYPE II DIABETES

Also known as non-insulin-dependent diabetes. The most common form of diabetes; injections of insulin are not necessary.

UNIVERSAL SCREENING

A screen or test which is applied to all or almost all persons within a given population, for instance hearing screening in schools.

UNREALISTIC OPTIMISM

A name given to the view that some people have that things will be better than they are statistically likely to be and that illnesses happen to 'other people'.

VALIDITY

In psychometrics, a term used to describe the extent to which a test actually assesses that which it purports to.

VISUAL ANALOGUE SCALE

A scale where people are asked to respond to a statement and do so by placing a mark along a line from two extremes, such as from 'Agree Totally' to 'Disagree Totally'. The measure of strength of response is given by the distance the mark is made along the line.

References

Abraham, C. and Sheeran, P. (1994). Modelling and modifying young hetero-sexuals' HIV preventive behaviour: a review of theories, findings and educational implications. *Patient Education and Counselling,* **23**, 173–86.

Adler, N.E., David, H.P., Major, B.N., Roth, S.H., Russo, N.F. and Wyatt, G.E. (1990). Psychological responses after abortion. *Science,* **248**, 41–4.

Aiken, L.S., West, S.G., Woodward, C.K. and Reno, R. (1994). Health beliefs and compliance with mammography screening recommendations in asymptomatic women. *Health Psychology,* **13**, 122–9.

Aikens, J.E., Kiolbasa, T.A. and Sobel, R. (1997). Psychological predictors of glycemic change with relaxation training in non-insulin dependent diabetes mellitus. *Psychotherapy and Psychosomatics,* **66**, 302–6.

Ajzen, I. (1985). From intentions to action: a theory of planned behavior. In J. Kuhl and J. Beckman (eds), *Action Control: from Cognitions to Behaviors.* New York: Springer.

Ajzen, I. (1988). *Attitudes, Personality and Behavior.* Milton Keynes: Open University Press.

Ajzen, I. (1991). The theory of planned behavior. *Organizational Behavior and Human Decision Processes,* **50**, 179–211.

Allison, D.B., Heshka, S., Neale, M.C., Lykken, D.T. and Heymsfield, S.B. (1994). A genetic analysis of relative weight among 4,020 twin pairs, with an emphasis on sex effects. *Health Psychology,* **13**, 362–5.

Antonovsky, A. and Hartman, H. (1974). Delay in the detection of cancer: a review. *Health Education Monographs,* **2**, 98–128.

Baillie, C., Smith, J., Hewison, J. and Mason, G. (2000). Ultrasound screening for chromosomal abnormality: Women's reactions to false positive results. *British Journal of Health Psychology,* **5**, 377–94.

Bakker, A.B., Buunk, B.P., Siero, F.W. and Van den Eijnden, R.J. (1997). Application of a modified health belief model to HIV preventive behavioral intentions among gay and bisexual men. *Psychology and Health,* **12**, 481–92.

Barber, T.X. (1982). Hypnosuggestive procedures in the treatment of clinical pain: implications for theories of hypnosis and suggestive therapy. In T. Millon, C. Green and R.B. Meagher (eds), *Handbook of Clinical Health Psychology.* New York: Plenum Press.

Becker, M.H. and Maiman, L.A. (1975). Sociobehavioural determinants of compliance with health and medical care recommendations. *Medical Care,* **13,** 10–24.

Becker, M.H., Maiman, L.A., Kirscht, J.P., Haefner, D.P. and Drachman, R.H. (1977). The health belief model and prediction of dietary compliance: A field experiment. *Journal of Health and Social Behaviour,* **18,** 348–66.

Beecher, H. (1946). Pain in men wounded in battle. *Bulletin of the United States Medical Department,* **5,** 445–54.

Beecher, H.K. (1956). Relationship of significance of wound to pain experienced. *Journal of the American Medical Association,* **161,** 1609–13.

Bennett, P. (2000). *Introduction to Clinical Health Psychology.* Buckingham: Open University Press.

Bennett, P. and Clatworthy, J. (1999). Smoking cessation during pregnancy: testing a psycho-biological model. *Psychology, Health and Medicine,* **4,** 319–26.

Berk, L.E. (2000). *Child Development, Fifth Edition.* Boston: Allyn and Bacon.

Berkman, L.F. and Syme, S.L. (1979). Social networks, host resistance, and mortality: a nine-year follow-up study of Alameda County residents. *American Journal of Epidemiology,* **109,** 186–204.

Bibace, R. and Walsh, M.E. (1979). Developmental stages in children's conceptions of illness. In G.C. Stone, F. Cohen and N.E. Adler (eds), *Health Psychology – A Handbook.* San Francisco: Jossey-Bass.

Blair, A. (1993). Social class and the contextualisation of illness experience. In A.Radley (ed.), *Worlds of Illness: Biographical and cultural perspectives on health and disease.* London: Routledge.

Booth, R., Koester, S., Brewster, J.T., Weibel, W.W. and Fritz, R.B. (1991). Intravenous drug users and AIDS: risk behaviors. *American Journal of Drug and Alcohol Abuse,* **17,** 337–53.

Bray, S.R., Gyurcsik, N.C., Culos-Reed, S.N., Dawson, K.A. and Martin, K.A. (2001). An exploratory investigation of the relationship between proxy efficacy, self-efficacy and exercise attendance. *Journal of Health Psychology,* **6,** 425–34.

Burroughs, W.S. (1956). Letter from a master addict to dangerous drugs. *British Journal of Addiction,* **53.**

Burroughs, W.S. (1977). *Junky.* New York: Penguin.

Butler, C. and Steptoe, A. (1986). Placebo responses: an experimental study of psychophysiological processes in asthmatic volunteers. *British Journal of Clinical Psychology,* **25,** 173–83.

Butler, C.C. and Evans, M. (1999). The 'heartsink' patient revisited. *British Journal of General Practice,* **49,** 230–3.

Cameron, L.D. (1997). Screening for Cancer: Illness Perceptions and Illness Worry. In K.J. Petrie and J.A. Weinman (eds), *Perceptions of Health and Illness.* Amsterdam: Harwood Academic.

Cannon, W.B. (1927). The James-Lange theory of emotions: a critical examination and an alternative. *American Journal of Psychology*, **39**, 106–24.

Cappell, H. and Greeley, J. (1987). Alcohol and tension reduction: an update on research and theory. In H.T. Blane and K.E. Leonard (eds), *Psychological Theories of Drinking and Alcoholism*. New York: Guilford Press.

Carroll, D. and Davey Smith, G. (1997). Health and socio-economic position: A commentary. *Journal of Health Psychology*, **2**, 275–82.

Carroll, D. and Niven, C.A. (1993). Gender, Health and Stress. In C. Niven and D. Carroll (eds), *The Health Psychology of Women*. Chur, Switzerland: Harwood Academic.

Cavelaars, A.E.J.M., Kunst, A.E. and Mackenbach, J.P. (1997). Socio-economic differences in risk factors for morbidity and mortality in the European Community. *Journal of Health Psychology*, **2**, 353–72.

Champion, V. and Miller, T. (1996). Predicting mammography utilization through model generation. *Psychology, Health and Medicine*, **1**, 273–83.

Cho, C. and Cassidy, D. (1994). Parallel processes for workers and their clients in chronic bereavement resulting from HIV. *Death Studies*, **18**, 273–92.

Clare, A.W. (1998). Psychological medicine. In P. Kumar and M. Clark (eds), *Clinical Medicine, Fourth Edition*. Edinburgh: W.B. Saunders.

Cohen, S., Tyrrell, D. and Smith, A. (1993). Negative life events, perceived stress, negative affect, and susceptibility to the common cold. *Journal of Personality and Social Psychology*, **64**, 131–40.

Cornwell, J. (1984). *Hard-Earned Lives: Accounts of Health and Illness from East London*. London: Tavistock.

Cronbach, L.J. (1951). Coefficient alpha and the internal structure of tests. *Psychometrika*, **22**, 293–6.

Crossley, M.L. (2000). *Rethinking Health Psychology*. Buckingham: Open University Press.

Croyle, R.T., Sun, Y.-C. and Hart, M. (1997). Processing Risk Factor Information: Defensive Biases in Health-Related Judgments and Memory. In K.J. Petrie and J.A. Weinman (eds), *Perceptions of Health and Illness*. Amsterdam: Harwood Academic.

Dakof, G.A. and Taylor, S.E. (1990). Victims' perceptions of social support: what is helpful from whom? *Journal of Personality and Social Psychology*, **58**, 80–9.

Davis, A., Bamford, J., Wilson, I., Ramkalawan, T., Forshaw, M. and Wright, S. (1997). A critical review of the role of neonatal hearing screening in the detection of congenital hearing impairment. *Health Technology Assessment*, **1**.

Davis, H. and Fallowfield, L. (1994). *Counselling and Communication in Healthcare*. Chichester: John Wiley.

De Craen, A.J.M., Roos, P.J., de Vries, A.L. and Kleijnen, J. (1996). Effect of colour of drugs: systematic review of perceived effect of drugs and of their effectiveness. *British Medical Journal*, **313**, 1624–6.

de Montigny, J. (1993). Distress, stress and solidarity in palliative care. *Omega: Journal of Death and Dying*, 27, 5–15.

Derogatis, L.R., Abeloff, M.D. and Melisaratos, N. (1979). Psychological coping mechanisms and survival time in metastatic breast cancer. *Journal of the American Medical Association*, 242, 1504–8.

Dunkel-Schetter, C., Feinstein, L., Taylor, S.E. and Falke, R (1992). Patterns of coping with cancer and their correlates. *Health Psychology*, 11, 79–87.

Duxbury, J. (2000). *Difficult Patients*. Oxford: Butterworth-Heinemann.

Egger, G., Fitzgerald, W., Frape, G., Monaem, A., Rubinstein, P., Tyler, C. and McKay, B. (1983). Results of large scale media antismoking campaign in Australia: North Coast 'Quit for Life' programme. *British Medical Journal*, 287, 1125–8.

Eiser, C. and Twamley, S. (1999). Talking to Children about Health and Illness. In M. Murray and K. Chamberlain (eds), *Qualitative Health Psychology*. London: Sage.

Elian, M. and Dean, G. (1985). To tell or not to tell the diagnosis of multiple sclerosis. *The Lancet*, 2, 27–8.

Ernst, E. and Resch, K.L. (1995). Concept of true and perceived placebo effects. *British Medical Journal*, 311, 551–3.

Eve, A., Smith, A.M. and Tebbit, P. (1997). Hospice and palliative care in the UK 1994–1995, including a summary of trends 1990–1995. *Palliative Medicine*, 11, 31–43.

Eysenck, H.J. (1973). Personality and the maintenance of the smoking habit. In W.L. Dunn (ed.), *Smoking Behavior: Motives and Incentives*. New York: Wiley.

Faber, J., Azzugnuni, M., Di Romana, S. and Vanhaeverbeek, M. (1991). [Letter] Fatal confusion between 'Losec' and 'Lasix', *The Lancet*, 337, 1286–7.

Feldman, P.E. (1956). The personal element in psychiatric research. *American Journal of Psychiatry*, 113, 52–4.

Ferguson, E. (1996). Hypochondriacal concerns: the roles of raw and calibrated medical knowledge. *Psychology, Health and Medicine*, 1, 315–18.

Festinger, L. (1957). *A Theory of Cognitive Dissonance*. Stanford: Stanford University Press.

Fine, P. (2000). Search for AIDS vaccine turns to brothels. *Times Higher Educational Supplement*, February 11.

Fiore, M.C., Smith, S.S., Jorenby, D.E. and Baker, T.B. (1994). The effectiveness of the nicotine patch for smoking cessation: a meta-analysis. *Journal of the American Medical Association*, 271, 1940–7.

Firth, S. (2000). Approaches to death in Hindu and Sikh communities in Britain. In D. Dickenson, M. Johnson and J.S. Katz (eds), *Death, Dying and Bereavement*. London: Sage/Open University.

Fisher, W.A. (1984). Predicting contraceptive behaviour among university men: the role of emotions and behavioural intentions. *Journal of Applied Social Psychology*, 14, 104–23.

Flesch, R.P. (1951). *How to Test Readability*. New York: Harper and Row.

Fletcher, D. (1997). Measles puts GPs' diagnosis on the spot. *The Daily Telegraph*, January 8th.

Flowers, P., Hart, G. and Marriott, C. (1999). Constructing sexual health: gay men and 'risk' in the context of a public sex environment. *Journal of Health Psychology*, **4**, 483–95.

Foley, F.J., Flannery, J., Graydon, D., Flintoft, G. *et al* (1995). AIDS palliative care: challenging the palliative paradigm. *Journal of Palliative Care*, **11**, 19–22.

Folkman, S., Lazarus, R.S., Dunkel-Schetter, C., DeLongis, A. and Gruen, R.J. (1986). Dynamics of a stressful encounter: cognitive appraisal, coping, and encounter outcomes. *Journal of Personality and Social Psychology*, **50**, 992–1003.

Foster, G.D., Wadden, T.A., Kendall, P.C., Stunkard, A.J. and Vogt, R.A. (1996). Psychological effects of weight loss and regain: a prospective study. *Journal of Consulting and Clinical Psychology*, **64**, 752–7.

Frankenhaeuser, M. (1975). Sympathetic adrenomedullary activity behavior and the psychosocial environment. In P.H. Venables and M.J. Christie (eds), *Research in Psychophysiology*. New York: Wiley.

French, K., Porter, A.M.D., Robinson, S.E., McCallum, F.R., Howie, J.G.R. and Roberts, M.M. (1982). Attendance at a breast screening clinic: a problem of administration or attitudes. *British Medical Journal*, **285**, 617–20.

French, S.A. and Jeffery, R.W. (1994). Consequences of dieting to lose weight: effects on physical and mental health. *Health Psychology*, **13**, 195–212.

Freudenberger, H.J. (1974). Staff burn-out. *Journal of Social Issues*, **30**, 159–65.

Friedman, M. and Rosenman, R.H. (1959). Association of specific overt behaviour pattern with blood and cardiovascular findings. *Journal of the American Medical Association*, **169**, 1286–97.

Friedman, M. and Rosenman, R.H. (1974). *Type A Behavior and Your Heart*. New York: Knopf.

Friedson, E. (1960). Client control and medical practice. *American Journal of Sociology*, **65**, 374–82.

Gale, E.A.M. and Anderson, J.V. (1998). Diabetes mellitus and other disorders of metabolism. In P. Kumar and M. Clark (eds), *Clinical Medicine, Fourth Edition*. Edinburgh: W.B. Saunders.

Garner, D.M. and Wooley, S.C. (1991). Confronting the failure of behavioral and dietary treatments for obesity. *Clinical Psychology Review*, **11**, 729–80.

Gehlert, S. (1996). Attributional style and locus of control in adults with epilepsy. *Journal of Health Psychology*, **4**, 469–77.

General Household Survey (1999). London: Office of Population Censuses and Surveys.

Gerbert, B. (1984). Perceived likeability and competence of simulated patients:

influence on physicians' management plans. *Social Science and Medicine,* **18**, 1053–60.

Gijsbers, K and Niven, C.A. (1993). Women and the Experience of Pain. In C.A. Niven and D. Carroll (eds), *The Health Psychology of Women.* Chur, Switzerland: Harwood Academic.

Gilley, J. (2000). Intimacy and terminal care. In D. Dickenson, M. Johnson and J.S. Katz (eds), *Death, Dying and Bereavement.* London: Sage/Open University.

Goolkasian, P. (1985). Phase and sex effects in pain perception: A critical review. *Psychology of Women Quarterly,* **9**, 15–28.

Gourlay, S.G., Forbes, A., Marriner, T., Pethica, D. and McNeil, J.J. (1994). Prospective study of factors predicting outcome of transdermal nicotine treatment in smoking cessation. *British Medical Journal,* **309**, 842–6.

Graham, H. (1998). Health at risk: poverty and national health strategies. In L. Doyal (ed.), *Women and Health Services.* Buckingham: Open University Press.

Grande, G.E., Todd, C.J. and Barclay, S.I.G. (1997). Support needs in the last year of life: patient and carer dilemmas. *Palliative Medicine,* **11**, 202–8.

Greer, S. (1991). Psychological response to cancer and survival. *Psychological Medicine,* **21**, 40–9.

Hadlow, J. and Pitts, M. (1991). The understanding of common health terms by doctors, nurses and patients. *Social Science and Medicine,* **32**, 193–6.

Hamburg, B.A. and Inoff, G.E. (1982). Relationship between behavioral factors and diabetic control in children and adolescents: a camp study. *Psychosomatic Medicine,* **44**, 321–9.

Hamer, D. and Copeland, P. (2000). *Living with Our Genes.* London: Pan.

Hampson, S. E. (1997). Illness Representations and the Self-Management of Diabetes. In K.J. Petrie and J.A. Weinman (eds), *Perceptions of Health and Illness.* Amsterdam: Harwood Academic.

Helman, C. (1995). Feed a cold, starve a fever. In B. Davey, A. Gray and C. Seale (eds), *Health and Disease: A Reader, Second Edition.* Buckingham: Open University Press.

Henderson, B.J. and Maguire, B.T. (1998). Lay representations of genetic disease, and predictive testing. *Journal of Health Psychology,* **3**, 233–41.

Herman, C.P. and Mack, D. (1975). Restrained and unrestrained eating. *Journal of Personality,* **43**, 647–60.

Hillhouse, J.J. and Adler, C.M. (1996). Evaluating a simple model of work stress, burnout, affective and physical symptoms in hospital nurses. *Psychology, Health and Medicine,* **1**, 297–306.

Hinton, J. (1999). The progress of awareness and acceptance of dying assessed in cancer patients and their caring relatives. *Palliative Medicine,* **13**, 19–35.

Hogbin, B. and Fallowfield, L.J. (1989). Getting it taped: the 'bad news' consultation with cancer patients. *British Journal of Hospital Medicine,* **41**, 330–3.

Holm, S. and Evans, M. (1996). Product names, proper claims? More ethical issues in the marketing of drugs. *British Medical Journal,* 313, 1627–9.

Holmes, D.S. (1984). Meditation and somatic arousal reduction: a review of the experimental evidence. *American Psychologist,* 39, 1–10.

Holmes, T.H. and Rahe, R.H. (1967). The Social Readjustment Rating Scale. *Journal of Psychosomatic Research,* 11, 213–18.

Hope, P. and Forshaw, M.J. (1999). Assessment of psychological distress is important in patients presenting with low back pain. *Physiotherapy,* 85, 563–70.

Houston, B.K. and Vavak, R.C. (1991). Hostility: developmental factors, psychosocial correlates and health behaviors. *Health Psychology,* 10, 9–17.

Hyyppae, M.T., Alaranta, H., Hurme, M., Nykvist, F. and Lahtel, K. (1988). Gender differences in psychological and cortisol responses to distress: a five-year follow-up of patients with back pain. *Stress Medicine,* 4, 117–21.

Istvan, J. and Matarazzo, J.D. (1984). Tobacco, alcohol, and caffeine use: a review of their interrelationships. *Psychological Bulletin,* 95, 301–26.

Jackson, C. and Lindsay, S. (1995). Reducing anxiety in new dental patients by means of a leaflet. *British Dental Journal,* 179, 163–7.

Jackson, R., Scragg, R. and Beaglehole, R. (1991). Alcohol consumption and risk of coronary heart disease. *British Medical Journal,* 303, 211–16.

Jacobsen, P.B., Bovbjerg, D.H. and Redd, W.H. (1993). Anticipatory anxiety in patients receiving cancer chemotherapy. *Health Psychology,* 12, 469–75.

Jeffery, R. (1979). Normal rubbish: deviant patients in casualty departments. *Sociology of Health and Illness,* 1, 90–108.

Jensen, M.P. and Karoly, P. (1991). Motivation and expectancy factors in symptom perception: a laboratory study of the placebo effect. *Psychosomatic Medicine,* 53, 144–52.

Jessor, R. and Jessor, S.L. (1977). *Problem behavior and psychosocial development: a longitudinal study of youth.* New York: Academic Press.

Johnson, S., Knight, R., Marmer, D.J. and Steele, R.W. (1981). Immune deficiency in fetal alcohol syndrome. *Pediatric Research,* 15, 908–11.

Johnston, M. (1996). Models of disability. *The Psychologist,* 9, 205–10.

Johnston, M. (1997). Representations of Disability. In K.J. Petrie and J.A. Weinman (eds), *Perceptions of Health and Illness,* Amsterdam: Harwood Academic.

Judd, D. (2000). Communicating with dying children. In D. Dickenson, M. Johnson and J.S. Katz (eds), *Death, Dying and Bereavement, Second Edition.* London: Sage/Open University.

Kalichman, S.C., Nachimson, D., Cherry, C. and Williams, E. (1998). AIDS treatment advances and behavioral prevention setbacks: preliminary assessment of reduced perceived threat of HIV-AIDS. *Health Psychology,* 17, 546–50.

Kane, B. (1979). Children's concepts of death. *Journal of Genetic Psychology,* 134, 141–53.

Kanner, A.D., Coyne, I.C., Schaefer, C. and Lazarus, R.S. (1981). Comparison of two modes of stress measurement: daily hassles and uplifts versus major life events. *Journal of Behavioral Medicine*, **4**, 1–39.

Kanvil, N. and Umeh, K.F. (2000). Lung cancer and cigarette use: cognitive factors, protection motivation and past behaviour. *British Journal of Health Psychology*, **5**, 235–48.

Kastenbaum, R. (2000). *The Psychology of Death, Third Edition*. London: Free Association Books.

Kawachi, I., Colditz, G.A. and Stone, C.B. (1994). Does coffee drinking increase the risk of coronary heart disease? Results from a meta-analysis. *British Heart Journal*, **72**, 269–75.

Keesey, R.E. (1980). The regulation of body weight: a set point analysis. In A.J. Stunkard (ed.), *Obesity*. Philadelphia: Saunders.

Kelleher, D. (1988). Coming to terms with diabetes: coping strategies and non-compliance. In R. Anderson and M. Bury (eds), *Living with Chronic Illness*. London: Allen and Unwin.

Kellner, R. (1985). Functional somatic systems and hypochondriasis. *Archives of General Psychiatry*, **42**, 821–33.

Kent, G. and Croucher, R. (1998). *Achieving Oral Health: The Social Context of Dental Care, Third Edition*. Oxford: Wright.

Kessler, R.C., Kendler, K.S., Heath, A.C., Neale, M.C. and Eaves, L.J. (1992). Social support, depressed mood, and adjustment to stress: a genetic epidemiological investigation. *Journal of Personality and Social Psychology*, **62**, 257–72.

Kiernan, P.J. and Isaacs, J.B. (1981). Use of drugs by the elderly. *Journal of the Royal Society of Medicine*, **74**, 196–200.

Killen, J.D., Robinson, T.N., Haydel, K.F., Hayward, C., Wilson, D.M., Hammer, L.D., Litt, I.F. and Taylor, C.B. (1997). Prospective study of risk factors for the initiation of cigarette smoking. *Journal of Consulting and Clinical Psychology*, **65**, 1011–16.

Kobasa, S.C. (1979). Stressful life events, personality, and health: an inquiry into hardiness. *Journal of Personality and Social Psychology*, **37**, 1–11.

Korsch, B.M. and Negrete, V. (1972). Doctor-patient communication. *Scientific American*, **227**, 66–74.

Koutantji, M., Pearce, S.A. and Oakley, D.A. (2000). Cognitive processing of pain-related words and psychological adjustment in high and low pain frequency participants. *British Journal of Health Psychology*, **5**, 275–88.

Kübler-Ross, E. (1969). *On death and dying*. New York: Macmillan.

Lando, H.A. (1977). Successful treatment of smokers with a broad-spectrum behavioral approach. *Journal of Consulting and Clinical Psychology*, **45**, 361–6.

Langewitz, W., Wossmer, B., Iseli, J. and Berger, W. (1997). Psychological and metabolic improvement after an outpatient teaching program for functional intensified insulin therapy. *Diabetes Research and Clinical Practice*, **37**, 157–64.

Lau, R.R. and Ware, J.E. (1981). Refinements in the measurement of health-specific locus-of-control beliefs. *Medical Care,* 19, 1147–58.

Lazarus, R. (1966). *Psychological Stress and the Coping Process.* New York: McGraw-Hill.

Leenaars, P.E.M., Rombouts, R. and Kok, G. (1993). Sexual medical care for a sexually transmitted disease: determinants of delay-behavior. *Psychology and Health,* 8, 17–32.

Levenson, H. (1974). Multidimensional locus of control in psychiatric patients. *Journal of Consulting and Clinical Psychology,* 41, 397–404.

Leventhal, H. and Avis, N. (1976). Pleasure, addiction, and habit: factors in verbal report or factors in smoking behavior? *Journal of Abnormal Psychology,* 85, 478–88.

Leventhal, H. and Cleary, P.D. (1980). The smoking problem: a review of research and theory in behavioral risk modification. *Psychological Bulletin,* 88, 370–405.

Leventhal, H., Meyer, D. and Nerenz, D. (1980). The common sense representation of illness danger. In S. Rachman (ed.), *Medical Psychology, Vol. 2.* New York: Pergamon.

Leventhal, H., Easterling, D.V., Coons, H., Luchterhand, C. and Love, R.R. (1986). Adaptation to chemotherapy treatments. In B. Anderson (ed.), *Women with Cancer.* New York: Springer Verlag.

Leventhal, H., Benyamini, Y., Brownlee, S., Diefenbach, M., Leventhal, E.A., Patrick-Miller, L. and Robitaille, C. (1997). Illness Representations: Theoretical Foundations. In K.J. Petrie and J.A. Weinman (eds) *Perceptions of Health and Illness.* Amsterdam: Harwood Academic.

Levine, F.M. and De Simone, L.L. (1991). The effects of experimenter gender on pain report in male and female subjects. *Pain,* 44, 69–72.

Lewis, V.J. and Blair, A.J. (1993). Women, Food and Body Image. In C.A. Niven and D. Carroll (eds), *The Health Psychology of Women.* Chur, Switzerland: Harwood Academic.

Ley, P. (1989). Improving patients' understanding, recall, satisfaction and compliance. In A.K. Broome (ed.), *Health Psychology.* London: Chapman and Hall.

Ley, P. (1997). Compliance among patients. In A. Baum, S. Newman, J. Weinman, R. West and C. McManus (eds), *Cambridge Handbook of Psychology, Health and Medicine.* Cambridge: Cambridge University Press.

Likert, R. (1952). A technique for the development of attitude scales. *Educational and Psychological Measurement,* 12, 313–15.

Lindemann, C. (1977). Factors affecting the use of contraception in the nonmarital context. In R. Gemme and C.C. Wheeler (eds), *Progress in Sexology.* New York: Plenum Press.

Lipton, J.A. and Marbach, J.J. (1984). Ethnicity and the pain experience. *Social Science and Medicine,* 19, 1279–98.

Longabaugh, R. and Morgenstern, J. (1999). Cognitive-behavioral coping-skills therapy for alcohol dependence: current status and future directions. *Alcohol Research and Health*, 23, 78–85.

Lowe, C.S. and Radius, S.M. (1982). Young adults' contraceptive practices: an investigation of influences. *Adolescence*, 22, 291–304.

MacIntyre, S. (1993). Gender differences in the perceptions of common cold symptoms. *Social Science and Medicine*, 36, 15–20.

Marks, G., Richardson, J.L. and Maldonado, N. (1991). Self disclosure of HIV infection to sexual partners. *American Journal of Public Health*, 81, 1321–3.

Marlatt, G.A. and Gordon, J.R. (1985). *Relapse Prevention*. New York: Guilford Press.

Marshall, J.R. and Funch, D.P. (1986). Gender and illness behaviour among colorectal cancer patients. *Women and Health*, 11, 67–82.

Marteau, T.M. (1989). Psychological costs of screening. *British Medical Journal*, 299, 527.

Marteau, T.M. (1993). Health-related screening: psychological predictors of uptake and impact. In S. Maes, H. Leventhal and M. Johnston (eds), *International Review of Health Psychology Volume II*. Chichester: Wiley.

Marteau, T.M. and Riordan, D.C. (1992). Staff attitudes to patients: the influence of causal attributions for illness. *British Journal of Clinical Psychology*, 31, 107–10.

Marteau, T.M., Slack, J., Kidd, J. and Shaw, R.W. (1992). Presenting a routine screening test in antenatal care: practice observed. *Public Health*, 106, 131–41.

Maslach, C. (1982). *Burnout: The Cost of Caring*. New York: Prentice-Hall.

Maslow, A.H. (1962). *Toward a psychology of being*. Princeton, NJ: Van Nostrand.

Mays, V.M. and Cochran, S.D. (1988). Issues in the perception of AIDS risk and risk reduction activities by Black and Hispanic/Latina women. *American Psychologist*, 43, 949–57.

Mazzulo, J.M., Lasagna, L. and Griner, P. (1974). Variation in interpretation of prescription instructions. *Journal of the American Medical Association*, 227, 29–31.

McAvoy, B.R. and Raza, R. (1988). Asian women: (i) Contraceptive knowledge, attitudes and usage, (ii) Contraceptive services and cervical cytology. *Health Trends*, 20, 11–17.

McCaul, K.D., Branstetter, A.D., Schroeder, D.M. and Glasgow, R.E. (1996). What is the relationship between breast cancer risk and mammography screening? A meta-analytic review. *Health Psychology*, 15, 423–9.

McCaul, K.D., Schroeder, D.M. and Reid, P.A. (1996). Breast cancer worry and screening: some prospective data. *Health Psychology*, 15, 430–3.

McManus, I.C., Lefford, F., Furnham, A.F., Shahidi, S. and Pincus, T. (1996). Career preference and personality differences in medical school applicants. *Psychology, Health and Medicine*, 1, 235–48.

Mechanic, D. (1978). *Medical Sociology, Second Edition*. New York: Free Press.

Medical Outcomes Trust (1993). *How to score the SF-36 Health Survey*. Boston, MA: Medical Outcomes Trust.

Meichenbaum, D. and Deffenbacher, J.L. (1988). Stress inoculation training. *Counseling Psychologist*, 16, 69–90.

Melzack, R. (1975). The McGill Pain Questionnaire: major properties and scoring methods. *Pain*, 1, 277–99.

Melzack, R. and Wall, P. (1982). *The Challenge of Pain*. Harmondsworth: Penguin.

Melzack, R. and Wall, P.D. (1965). Pain mechanisms: a new theory. *Science*, 150, 971–9.

Merikle, P.M. and Skanes, H.E. (1992). Subliminal self-help audiotapes: a search for placebo effects. *Journal of Applied Psychology*, 77, 772–6.

Miller, C.T. and Downey, K.T. (1999). A meta-analysis of heavyweight and self-esteem. *Journal of Consulting and Clinical Psychology*, 65, 448–52.

Miller, D., Green, J., Farmer, R. and Carroll, G. (1985). A 'pseudo-AIDS' syndrome following from a fear of AIDS. *British Journal of Psychiatry*, 146, 550.

Miller, T.Q., Smith, T.W., Turner C.W., Guijarro, M.L. and Hallet, A.J. (1996). A meta-analytic review of research on hostility and physical health. *Psychological Bulletin*, 119, 322–48.

Monjan, A.A. (1981). Stress and immunologic competence: Studies in animals. In R. Ader (ed.), *Psychoneuroimmunology*. New York: Academic Press.

Montgomery, J. (1997). *Health Care Law*. Oxford: Oxford University Press.

Mosbach, P. and Leventhal, H. (1988). Peer group identification and smoking: implications for intervention. *Journal of Abnormal Psychology*, 97, 238–45.

Mulatu, M.S. (1999). Perceptions of mental and physical illnesses in north-western Ethiopia: causes, treatments, and attitudes. *Journal of Health Psychology*, 4, 531–49.

Murray, M. and Chamberlain, K. (eds) (1999). *Qualitative Health Psychology: Theories and Methods*. London: Sage.

Napoleon, H. (1999). *Yuuyaraq*: The Way of the Human Being. In C. Samson (ed.), *Health Studies: A Critical and Cross-Cultural Reader*. Oxford: Blackwell.

Nekolaichuk, C.L. and Bruera, E. (1998). On the nature of hope in palliative care. *Journal of Palliative Care*, 14, 36–42.

Newton, J. (1995). The readability and utility of general dental practice patient information leaflets: an evaluation. *British Dental Journal*, 178, 329–32.

Nichols, K.A. (1993). *Psychological Care in Physical Illness, Second Edition*. London: Chapman and Hall.

Nolen-Hoeksema, S., McBride, A. and Larson, J. (1997). Rumination and psychological distress among bereaved partners. *Journal of Personality and Social Psychology*, 72, 855–62.

O'Leary, A.O. (1990). Stress, emotion, and human immune function. *Psychological Bulletin*, **108**, 363–82.

Oakley, A. (1980). *Women Confined*. Oxford: Martin Robertson.

Office of National Statistics. (1999). *Social Trends 29*. London: The Stationery Office.

Ogden, J. and Fox, P. (1994). An examination of the use of smoking for weight control in restrained and unrestrained eaters. *International Journal of Eating Disorders*, **16**, 177–86.

Orbell, S. and Sheeran, P. (1993). Health psychology and uptake of preventive health services: a review of 30 years' research on cervical screening. *Psychology and Health*, **8**, 417–33.

Parkes, C.M. (2000). Bereavement as a psychosocial transition: processes of adaptation to change. In D. Dickenson, M. Johnson and J.S. Katz (eds), *Death, Dying and Bereavement, Second Edition*. London: Sage/Open University.

Payne, S.A., Langley-Evans, A. and Hiller, R. (1996). Perceptions of a 'good' death: a comparative study of the views of hospice staff and patients. *Palliative Medicine*, **10**, 307–12.

Payne, S., Smith, P. and Dean, S. (1999). Identifying the concerns of informal carers in palliative care. *Palliative Medicine*, **13**, 37–44.

Pelham, B.W. (1999). *Conducting Experiments in Psychology – Measuring the Weight of Smoke*. Pacific Grove, CA: Brooks/Cole.

Pettingale, K.W., Morris, T., Greer, S. and Haybittle, J.L. (1985). Mental attitudes to cancer: an additional prognostic factor. *The Lancet*, **1**, 750.

Phoenix, A. (1989). Influences on previous contraceptive use/non-use in pregnant 16–19 year olds. *Journal of Reproductive and Infant Psychology*, **7**, 211–25.

Pomerleau, O.F. and Pomerleau, C.S. (1989). A biobehavioral perspective on smoking. In T. Ney and A. Gale (eds), *Smoking and Behavior*. Chichester: John Wiley.

Povey, R., Conner, M., Sparks, P., James, R. and Shepherd, R. (2000). Application of the Theory of Planned Behaviour to two dietary behaviours: Roles of perceived control and self-efficacy. *British Journal of Health Psychology*, **5**, 121–39.

Pridmore, P. and Bendelow, G. (1995). Images of health: exploring the beliefs of children using the 'draw and write' technique. *Health Education Journal*, **54**, 473–88.

Reeve, J., Owens, R.G. and Winship, I.M. (2000). Psychological impact of predictive testing for colonic cancer. *Journal of Health Psychology*, **5**, 99–108.

Rigby, K., Brown, M., Anganostou, P., Ross, M.W. *et al* (1989). Shock tactics to counter AIDS: the Australian experience. *Psychology and Health*, **3**, 145–59.

Rimer, B.K. (1992). Understanding the acceptance of mammography by women. *Annals of Behavioral Medicine*, **14**, 197–203.

Robb, N. and Smith, B. (1996). Anorexia and bulimia nervosa (the eating disorders): conditions of interest to the dental practitioner. *Journal of Dentistry*, **24**, 7–16.

Robson, C. (1993). *Real World Research – A Resource for Social Scientists and Practitioner–Researchers*. Oxford: Blackwell.

Roethlisberger, F.J. and Dickson, W.J. (1939). *Management and the worker*. Cambridge, MA: Harvard University Press.

Rogers, R.W. (1975). A protection motivation theory of fear appeals and attitude change. *Journal of Psychology*, **91**, 93–114.

Rogers, R.W. (1983). Cognitive and physiological processes in fear appeals and attitude change. A revised theory of protection motivation. In J.R. Cacioppo and R.E. Petty (eds), *Social Psychology: A Source Book*. New York: Guilford Press.

Rosenstock, I.M. (1966). Why people use health services. *Millbank Memorial Fund Quarterly*, **44**, 94–124.

Ross, M. and Olson, J.M. (1981). An expectancy attribution model of the effects of placebos. *Psychological Review*, **88**, 408–37.

Rotter, J.B. (1966). Generalized expectancies for internal versus external control of reinforcement. *Psychological Monographs*, **80** (1, Whole No. 609).

Sadler, M. (1997). Serum screening for Down's syndrome: how much do health professionals know? *British Journal of Obstetrics and Gynaecology*, **104**, 176–9.

Salkovskis, P.M. and Warwick, H.M.C. (1986). Morbid preoccupations, health anxiety and reassurance: a cognitive behavioural approach to hypochondriasis. *Behaviour Research and Therapy*, **24**, 597–602.

Salmon, P. (2000). *Psychology of Medicine and Surgery*. Chichester: John Wiley.

Salovey, P. and Birnbaum, D. (1989). Influence of mood on health-relevant cognitions. *Journal of Personality and Social Psychology*, **57**, 539–51.

Savage, R. and Armstrong, D. (1990). Effect of a general practitioner's consulting style on patient satisfaction: a controlled study. *British Medical Journal*, **301**, 968–70.

Schachter, S. (1977). Nicotine regulation in heavy and light smokers. *Journal of Experimental Psychology: General*, **106**, 5–12.

Schachter, S. (1982). Recidivism and self-cure of smoking and obesity. *American Psychologist*, **37**, 436–44.

Scheier, M.F. and Carver, C.S. (1985). Optimism, coping, and health: assessment and implications of generalized outcome expectancies. *Health Psychology*, **4**, 219–47.

Scheier, M.F., Carver, C.S. and Bridges, M.W. (1994). Distinguishing optimism from neuroticism (and trait anxiety, self-mastery, and self-esteem): a re-evaluation of the life orientation test. *Journal of Personality and Social Psychology*, **67**, 1063–78.

Scheier, M.F., Matthews, K.A., Owens, J., Magovern, G.J. *et al* (1989). Dispositional optimism and recovery from coronary artery bypass surgery: the beneficial effects on physical and psychological well-being. *Journal of Personality and Social Psychology*, 57, 1024–40.

Scheper-Hughes, N. (1999). Nervoso: Medicine, Sickness, and Human Needs. In C. Samson (ed.), *Health Studies: A Critical and Cross-Cultural Reader*. Oxford: Blackwell.

Schifter, D.E. and Ajzen, I. (1985). Intention, perceived control, and weight loss: an application of the theory of planned behavior. *Journal of Personality and Social Psychology*, 49, 843–51.

Schmidt, W. (1977). Cirrhosis and alcohol consumption: an epidemiological perspective. In G. Edwards and M. Grant (eds), *Alcoholism: New Knowledge and New Responses*. London: Croom Helm.

Schwarzer, R. (1992). Self-efficacy in the adoption and maintenance of health behaviors: Theoretical approaches and a new model. In R. Schwarzer (ed.), *Self-Efficacy: Thought Control of Action*. Washington, DC: Hemisphere.

Seidell, J.C and Rissenen, A.M. (1998). Time trends in world-wide prevalence of obesity. In G.A. Bray, C. Bouchard and W.P.T James (eds), *Handbook of Obesity*. New York: Marcel Dekker.

Shaffer, J.W., Graves, P.L., Swank, R.T. and Pearson, T.A. (1987). Clustering of personality traits in youth and the subsequent development of cancer in physicians. *Journal of Behavioral Medicine*, 10, 441–7.

Shapiro, A.K. (1964). Factors contributing to the placebo effect: their implications for psychotherapy. *American Journal of Psychotherapy*, 18, 73–88.

Sheeran, P. and Abraham, C. (1995). 'The Health Belief Model'. In M. Conner and P. Norman (eds), *Predicting Health Behaviour*. Buckingham: Open University Press.

Shiffman, S., Paty, J.A., Gnys, M., Kassel, J.D. and Elash, C. (1995). Nicotine withdrawal in chippers and regular smokers: subjective and cognitive effects. *Health Psychology*, 14, 301–9.

Shontz, F.C. (1975). *The Psychological Aspects of Physical Disease and Disability*. New York: Macmillan.

Siegel, K., Schrimshaw, E.W. and Dean, L. (1999). Symptom interpretation and medication adherence among late middle-age and older HIV-infected adults. *Journal of Health Psychology*, 4, 247–57.

Sinyor, D., Schwartz, J.G., Peronnet, F., Bisson, G. and Seraganian, P. (1983). Aerobic fitness level and reactivity to psychosocial stress. *Psychosomatic Medicine*, 45, 205–17.

Sissons Joshi, M. (1995). Lay explanations of the causes of diabetes in India and the UK. In I. Markova and R.M. Farr (eds), *Representations of health, illness and handicap*. Philadelphia: Harwood.

Sjöström, L. (1980). Fat cells and body weight. In A.J. Stunkard (ed.), *Obesity*. Philadelphia: Saunders.

Sklar, L.S and Anisman, H. (1981). Stress and cancer. *Psychological Bulletin,* 89, 369–406.

Sobo, E.J. (1993). Inner-city women and AIDS: the psycho-social benefits of unsafe sex. *Culture, Medicine and Psychiatry,* 17, 455–85.

Spinetta, J.J. (1974). The dying child's awareness of death: a review. *Psychological Bulletin,* 81, 256–60.

Spitzer, L. and Rodin, J. (1981). Human eating behaviour: a critical review of studies in normal weight and overweight individuals. *Appetite,* 2, 293–329.

Stacey, M. (1988). *The Sociology of Health and Healing.* London: Unwin Hyman.

Steed, L., Newman, S.P. and Hardman, S.M.C. (1999). An examination of the self-regulation model in atrial fibrillation. *British Journal of Health Psychology,* 4, 337–47.

Stein, Z.A. (1990). HIV prevention: the need for methods women can use. *American Journal of Public Health,* 80, 460–2.

Stoller, E.P. (1984). Self-assessments of health by the elderly: the impact of informal assistance. *Journal of Health and Social Behavior,* 25, 260–70.

Strauss, J., Muday, T., McNall, K. and Wong, M. (1997). Response Style Theory revisited: gender differences and stereotypes in rumination and distraction. *Sex Roles,* 36, 771–92.

Stroebe, W. (2000). *Social Psychology and Health, Second Edition.* Buckingham: Open University Press.

Suter, P.O., Schutz, Y. and Jequier, A. (1992). The effect of ethanol on fat storage in healthy subjects. *New England Journal of Medicine,* 326, 983–7.

Swinker, M., Arbogast, J.B. and Murray, S. (1993). Why do patients decline screening mammography? *Family Practice Research Journal,* 13, 165–70.

Tattersall, M.H., Butow, P.N., Griffin, A-M. and Dunn, S.M. (1994). The take-home message: patients prefer consultation audiotapes to summary letters. *Journal of Clinical Oncology,* 12, 1305–11.

Taylor, N.M., Hall, G.M. and Salmon, P. (1996). Patients' experiences of patient-controlled analgesia. *Anaesthesia,* 51, 525–8.

Taylor, S.E. (1983). Adjustment to threatening events: a theory of cognitive adaptation. *American Psychologist,* 38, 1161–73.

Taylor, S.E., Lichtman, R.R. and Wood, J.V. (1984). Attributions, beliefs about control, and adjustment to breast cancer. *Journal of Personality and Social Psychology,* 46, 489–502.

Teicher, M.H., Glod, C.A., Magnus, E., Harper, D., Benson, G., Krueger, K. and McGreenery, C.E. (1997). Circadian rest-activity disturbances in seasonal affective disorder. *Archives of General Psychiatry,* 54, 124–30.

Temoshok, L. (1987). Personality, coping style, emotion and cancer: toward an integrative model. *Social Science and Medicine,* 20, 833–40.

Temoshok, L., Sweet, D.M. and Zich, J.A. (1987). A three city comparison of the public's knowledge and attitudes about AIDS. *Psychology and Health,* 1, 43–60.

Thelin, T., McNeil, T.F., Aspegren-Jansson, E. and Sveger, T. (1985). Psychological consequences of neonatal screening for alpha-1–antitrypsin deficiency (ATD) – parental attitudes toward ATD-check-ups and parental recommendations regarding future screening. *Acta Paediatrica Scandinavica*, **74**, 841–7.

Tluczek, A., Mischler, E.H., Bowers, B., Peterson, N.M., Morris, M.E., Farrell, P.M., Bruns, W.T., Colby, H., McCarthy, C., Fost, N. and Carey, P. (1991). Psychological impact of false-positive results when screening for cystic fibrosis. *Pediatric Pulmonology Supplement*, **7**, 29–37.

Tluczek, A., Mischler, E.H., Farrell, P.M., Fost, N., Peterson, N.M., Carey, P., Bruns, W.T. and McCarthy, C. (1992). Parents' knowledge of neonatal screening and response to false-positive cystic fibrosis testing. *Journal of Developmental and Behavioral Pediatrics*, **13**, 181–6.

Totman, R.G. (1987). *The Social Causes of Illness*. London: Souvenir Press.

Toynbee, P. (1977). *Patients*. New York: Harcourt Brace.

Vernon, S.W., Laville, E.A. and Jackson, G.L. (1990). Participation in breast screening programs: a review. *Social Science and Medicine*, **30**, 1107–18.

Visintainer, M., Volpicelli, J. and Seligman, M. (1982). Tumor rejection in rats after inescapable or escapable shock. *Science*, **216**, 437–9.

Wald, N.J., Kennard, A., Hackshaw, A. and McGuire, A. (1997). Antenatal screening for Down's syndrome. *Journal of Medical Screening*, **4**, 181–246.

Waldron, E. (1976). Why do women live longer than men? *Journal of Human Stress*, **2**, 2–13.

Walker, L.S., Garber, J. and Greene, J.W. (1991). Somatization symptoms in pediatric abdominal pain patients: relation to chronicity of abdominal pain and parent somatization. *Journal of Abnormal Child Psychology*, **19**, 379–94.

Wallston, K.A. and Wallston, B.S. (1980). Health locus of control scales. In H. Lefcourt (ed.), *Advances and Innovations in Locus of Control Research*. New York: Academic Press.

Wallston, K.A., Wallston, B.S. and DeVellis, R. (1978). Development of the multidimensional health locus of control (MHLC) scales. *Health Education Monographs*, **6**, 160–70.

Walter, T., Littlewood, J. and Pickering, M. (2000). Death in the news: the public investigation of private emotion. In D. Dickenson, M. Johnson and J.S. Katz (eds), *Death, Dying and Bereavement, Second Edition*. London: Sage/Open University.

Wardle, J. and Beales, S. (1988). Control and loss of control over eating: an experimental investigation. *Journal of Abnormal Psychology*, **97**, 35–40.

Warwick, H.M.C. and Salkovskis, P.M. (1990). Hypochondriasis. *Behaviour Research and Therapy*, **28**, 105–17.

Watson, D. and Pennebaker, J.W. (1989). Health complaints, stress, and distress: Exploring the central role of negative affectivity. *Psychological Review*, **96**, 234–54.

Weinstein, N. (1984). Why it won't happen to me: Perceptions of risk factors and susceptibility. *Health Psychology,* **3**, 431–57.

Weinstein, N.D. (1982). Unrealistic optimism about susceptibility to health problems. *Journal of Behavioral Medicine,* **5**, 441–60.

Whitely, B.E. and Schofield, J.W. (1986). A meta-analysis of research on adolescent contraceptive use: population and environment. *Behavioral and Social Issues,* **8**, 173–203.

Wiens, A.N. and Menustik, C.E. (1983). Treatment outcome and patient characteristics in an aversion therapy program for alcoholism. *American Psychologist,* **38**, 1089–96.

Wilkinson, S. (1991). Factors which influence how nurses communicate with cancer patients. *Journal of Advanced Nursing,* **16**, 677–88.

Williams, S. (2001). 'Barebacking', HIV risk and health promotion. *The Psychologist,* **14**, 90.

Willis, P.E. (1993). The Expressive Style of a Motor-bike Culture. In A. Beattie, M. Gott, L. Jones and M. Sidell (eds), *Health and Wellbeing: a Reader.* Basingstoke: Macmillan/Open University Press.

Woods, S., Natterson, J. and Silverman, J. (1966). Medical students' disease: hypochondriasis in medical students. *Journal of Medical Education,* **41**, 785–90.

Wright, C.J. and Mueller, C.B. (1995). Screening mammography and public health policy: the need for perspective. *The Lancet,* **346**, 29–32.

Wurster, C., Weinstein, P. and Cohen, A. (1979). Communication patterns and pedodontics. *Perceptual and Motor Skills,* **48**, 159–66.

Zimba, C.G. and Buggie, S.E. (1993). An experimental study of the placebo effect in African traditional medicine. *Behavioral Medicine,* **19**, 103–9.

Zola, I.K. (1966). Culture and symptoms: an analysis of patients' presenting complaints. *American Sociological Review,* **31**, 615–30.

Name Index

Subject Index